Praise for Thanks For My Kidn

"Beautifully honest, heartfelt and courageous."

Nicos Kessaris (consultant transplant surgeon)

"This heart-warming story explores the roller-coaster ride of emotion and anxiety of end-stage kidney failure from the perspective of someone who has lived through this life-changing event. This courageously honest and uplifting account will inform and educate both healthcare professionals and patients."

Rachel Hilton (consultant nephrologist)

"This is a great book sharing lived experience that will be invaluable to both women with kidney transplants and health care professionals."

Kate Bramham (consultant nephrologist)

"Kay has bravely reflected back on her personal kidney journey, which highlights the ups and downs that she faced and continues to face. She raises awareness of kidney disease and the importance of organ donation and transplantation. This brave account is an inspiring and informative read."

National Kidney Federation

I hope you enjoy reading my book!
Love Kay x

Thanks For My Kidney, Mum!

A young woman's journey through kidney
transplant surgery and life beyond

KAY ALLARDYCE

For my supportive parents,
Patrick Tomlinson and Linda Tomlinson,
who are always there for me no matter what.

For my one-in-a-million aunt, Lisa Kinsey.

For my super encouraging husband, Tim.

And lastly...

For my beautiful children, George and Rosealin,
who I love with all my heart.

Contents

Preface

IN 2007, I WAS DIAGNOSED with chronic kidney disease (CKD) – a devastating diagnosis that left me with feelings of despair and hopelessness. My future, once bright with promise and possibility, suddenly became uncertain and daunting. How was I supposed to plan for my future when I had no idea if I even had a future? Would I need a kidney transplant? Would I be able to marry and have children of my own? What if I became unable to work? These questions suddenly became very real as I faced the uncertainty of my diagnosis.

In the midst of my uncertainty was an overwhelming desire to educate myself about my illness and to help others facing CKD and possible kidney transplantation surgery. Many times, I tried to write about my experience but realised that the time just wasn't right. For me, self-reflection was like opening an old wound and was emotionally very painful. I found that burying the past was the easier option. Finally, with the love and encouragement of my wonderful husband, Tim, I found the courage and inner strength to write my story.

I've now had sixteen years living with CKD, and ten years post-transplant, the kidney of which I was very fortunate to receive from my mother. I am now a mother myself to two children, both born following my transplant.

I pray that my story offers useful information and can give hope to others facing a diagnosis of CKD or another chronic health disorder. I believe there is lots we can learn from others' lived experiences. For those who face the challenges of pregnancy and childbirth after a kidney transplant, I hope this book gives you hope and encouragement that, like me, it is possible.

Prologue

"IT'S JUST BAD LUCK, MY DEAR," the consultant remarked when I asked, "Why has this happened to me?"

My body was shivery, with clammy hands and a hot face. It was as though I had massively flunked an exam at school, never to be able to re-sit it. How was I going to explain this to my parents? Never wanting to let them down or disappoint them, I was always the Bs-or-above girl. I felt my face fall. In response to this, the consultant followed with "You're very lucky your body gave you symptoms at all. Many people have no warning signs until their kidneys are at the point of failure!"

Suddenly I didn't feel so lucky. It was nice to know that my body did something great, but all I felt was a massive sense of disappointment. Today was the beginning of a lifelong journey of treatment and monitoring.

God, I would gladly take a failing grade any day instead of this.

Part One

The Early Years

1
Tell-tale signs

I WAS TWENTY-FOUR YEARS OLD when I was diagnosed with chronic kidney disease, or CKD. The technical term for my disease is focal segmental glomerulosclerosis, or FSGS. I felt many things when I got the diagnosis, but what I felt the most was that I had been cheated. I had always tried to live a reasonably healthy lifestyle, eating sensibly and staying physically active. Now, I had been cursed with a life-altering disease.

I was a year out of university, where I had studied to become an osteopath and naturopath, trying to get work wherever I could. It was a pretty tough year emotionally, as all I wanted was to be busy, treating patients and keeping my hands and mind occupied, but all I had was spare time. I was low. I remember thinking, *I've got so much time on my hands. I could be unwell and coping with some health problem and still have time for work.* A very stupid thought, and one I will always regret.

I took a postgraduate acupuncture course, which recommended hepatitis B vaccination – a series of three injections given at specified intervals. The vaccine is given to prevent infection due to accidental blood exposure from the single-use acupuncture needles. After my first dose, terrible acne appeared on my back. I tried to treat the lesions with a natural sugar and lemon juice scrub which, as you can imagine, was very painful! As I know now, the skin is an indicator of the body's overall health. My skin tone was changing, and new hair growth looked frazzled and unhealthy. I had also noticed my urine had a different smell and had become frothy. I didn't have any pain when urinating, so it didn't concern me too much. I thought maybe the toilet bowl cleaner was reacting with my urine. I had the following two required hepatitis B injections without incident. A few uneventful months passed, and I didn't give much more thought to the skin and urinary symptoms.

Then the swelling started...

2

A wedding in Naples

IT WAS JULY 2007 AND I HAD travelled to Naples, Italy, for a wedding. Like most weddings abroad, the weather was hot and my flight was long. It involved lots of eating (seven courses, in fact!), drinking and sitting for long periods of time. I noticed that my feet and ankles felt tight in some strappy shoes I was wearing. Women's shoes are uncomfortable anyway, but these were doubly so due to the swelling.

I tried elevating and massaging my feet and legs, which didn't help at all. I would wake after a good night's sleep and see a slight improvement, but the 'puffiness' was there all the time. The ankle swelling just would not go. At this point I began to suspect a link between my skin and hair symptoms and my swollen ankles, and that the problem could be serious. As an osteopath, you would think I'd have made the connection sooner.

This went on for two weeks and, yes, I did bury my head in the sand. I had just finished my degree and had learned the importance of timely evaluation and intervention. I'm not sure why I waited so long to be evaluated. I suppose it was because I knew that something serious was going on and I didn't want to face it. Maybe I was hopeful that one day it would just be gone!

I was working in a clinic in Tonbridge at the time, with a very knowledgeable osteopath who had also been a GP for many years. I popped into his consulting room one afternoon in between seeing my own patients, just to ask his opinion regarding my ankles. He took one look at them and told me to get an emergency appointment with my GP. *TODAY!* He even telephoned me later to be sure I had one booked! That evening, I saw my GP, who immediately took my blood pressure and said it was sky high. She sent me off straight away to the blood pressure hypertension unit at St George's Hospital in Tooting. I started thinking about how I had felt over the last few weeks and recollected some nasty headaches too. I had ignored them, as I was whizzing around trying to work as much as possible to be able to pay off loans I had taken out for my osteopathy course. I attributed my headaches to stress and work.

3
Life-changing results

MY ORDEAL BEGAN AT ST GEORGE'S Hospital in Tooting, London. As the team took a blood specimen, I started sweating and then became light-headed. Little did I know that this would to be the first of hundreds of blood tests taken over the next fifteen years! The team immediately suspected I had kidney issues and began evaluating the markers measuring kidney function.

Simply put, my markers were a mess. My creatinine level was too high at 138umol/L (normal range for women is 45 to 90umol/L); my estimated glomerular filtration rate (eGFR) was 40 (normal should be 60 or higher); my cholesterol was 10.3mmol/L (above 7.8mmol/L is classified as very high); my albumin was low at 21g/L (normal is 35–55g/L).

Next, I was given a ridiculously small specimen cup to collect a urine sample for testing – again, the first of many ahead. Trying to keep the urine off my fingers while aiming it into the cup was quite comical, actually. My urine showed high levels of protein (proteinuria), and red blood cells (haematuria). No wonder my albumin was so low, considering 50–60% of it is composed of blood plasma protein. The protein was leaking through the kidneys and was being excreted in my urine.

Next on the list was an ultrasound scan of both kidneys. This showed enlargement of my kidneys – the right more so than the left, measuring 13.2cm. A normal-size kidney is about the size of your fist, approximately 10–12cm.

Finally, I was booked in for a kidney biopsy. When evaluating kidney function, the biopsy is the 'gold standard' of tests. The biopsy was uncomfortable but didn't take more than fifteen minutes. I was lying on my front and the part of my back between the lower ribs and pelvis was numbed. This is where the kidneys sit, deep on each side of the body. A long biopsy needle was inserted to take a piece of tissue from the kidney for examination at a histology laboratory. I could feel my heart beating and my blood pressure rising before the procedure, and my chest became tight from anxiety at what was happening. The team had to stabilise my blood pressure and wait for my chest tightness to subside. I just wanted to get on with it! Waiting was excruciating, as my mind was working overtime. I was so nervous, not knowing what to expect or what the outcome would show. Eventually, the team performed the biopsy. My overactive mind was visualising what was happening while feeling the prodding and poking. There was no pain, just some discomfort. Then the profuse sweating started again. I was afraid to look around or move until the consultant said I could. I had to lie down for about six hours following the biopsy due to the risk of bleeding and to prevent deep vein thrombosis, which is the formation and dislodging of blood clots. After adequate time in recovery, I was discharged to go home the same day.

I also went home with a diagnosis. I had stage 3 CKD, specifically focal segmental glomerulosclerosis, or FSGS. I had segmental sclerosis (or scarring) in the glomeruli, with some possible signs of IgA nephropathy. Both conditions are classified as autoimmune conditions that create scarring in the glomeruli. This scarring had greatly reduced the filtering capacity of both of my kidneys. I had no idea what this diagnosis meant.

But I knew that, as of today, my life would be forever changed.

4
Kidney function and FSGS

WHILE THE KIDNEYS HELP TO MAINTAIN many of the body's systems, the main function of the kidneys is to filter waste and toxic substances from the blood. The consultant explained FSGS to me as pockets of scarring in the kidneys. Under a microscope, each kidney has millions of tiny little filters called glomeruli that act much like a kitchen colander. Blood circulates into these, and the water-like part of the blood is filtered to create urine. Scarred glomeruli cannot function effectively as filters. 'Focal' and 'segmental' meant that not all the glomeruli were affected, and only specific parts of those glomeruli were affected. The short version? The little filters in my kidneys were scarred beyond repair and could no longer function as filters to remove waste products and toxins from my body.

I really wanted to know what had caused my disease, and to hear that the cause was "unknown" and "bad luck" was a bitter pill to swallow. The nephrologist at the time said that sometimes there are no signs or symptoms until you're in renal failure and in need of dialysis. Maybe in a way I *was* lucky! I sure didn't feel that way. Why me? Maybe my nights of heavy drinking as a student had taken their toll, but none of my other friends were facing anything like this!

Had it been the hepatitis B vaccine that sparked something off? To this day, it's still hard to accept that my disease was simply caused by "bad luck". Like so many other autoimmune-type conditions, there is a lot of research to be done to determine a possible cause.

The diagnosis of FSGS is usually sub-grouped into 'primary' (as was mine), which means that the disease happens on its own due to an unknown cause, or the other sub-group is 'secondary', which means the disease is caused by another medical condition. Some possible causes are sickle cell anaemia, viruses (such as HIV), urine backing up in the kidneys, kidney defects from birth, obesity and obstructive sleep apnoea.

5
Treatment in the first six months

THE MANAGEMENT PLAN OF MY KIDNEY disease in the early days was to control my blood pressure and reduce the proteinuria (protein leaking into my urine) as much as possible. I was also put on a low sodium and low potassium diet. My medications consisted of ramipril (an angiotensin-converting enzyme inhibitor), and amlodipine (a calcium channel blocker). Both were to help relax and dilate the blood vessels, which reduce the blood pressure. Furosemide, a diuretic, was prescribed to decrease the swelling. This medication decreases the amount of excess water in the body by increasing the amount of urine you excrete. Atorvastatin was prescribed to help lower my cholesterol.

The anti-coagulant drug warfarin was prescribed to prevent the formation of blood clots. I am glad to say I took warfarin for only a short time. This medication was necessary due to very low albumin levels (a type of blood protein). This was a consequence of the protein lost through my poorly filtering kidneys. It was a tricky business trying to keep my international normalised ratio

(INR) at the correct level. This test measures the time it takes for your blood to clot. The INR must be maintained within the optimal range. If not, the blood may become too thin, causing uncontrolled bleeding, or too thick, which can cause a stroke or heart attack. Lots of different foods and drinks seemed to affect the INR. At this stage I was at the hospital a few times a week having my blood tested until my INR stabilised. I seemed to be the youngest person having this test done (I did get some very inquisitive looks!). My levels eventually improved enough to come off the warfarin, which was a massive relief. Attending appointments took so much of my time, and parking at the various hospitals was so expensive! I would try and see a few patients in one practice, shoot off to the hospital a few miles down the road to get my bloods done, then go on to a different practice to see another patient seeking osteopathy treatment. Life was suddenly busy, but not necessarily for the reasons I had hoped for at the start of my career.

6
The dreaded low sodium/ low potassium diet

A MAJOR ADJUSTMENT FOR ME WAS the low potassium diet. It just seemed so opposite to all I had learned about healthy diets as part of my naturopathic studies. Boiling all my vegetables and limiting them to only two a day alongside just two portions of fruit felt so wrong to me. I had to avoid high potassium foods like bananas and avocados, and stop snacking on dried fruit, nuts and seeds, all of which I really enjoyed. So what was I allowed to snack on instead? Worst of all was giving up chocolate, which I loved to eat occasionally as a little treat! Also banned were fruit juices and ice cream (and it was the middle of the summer!!). Lower potassium food choices that were suggested just seemed so counterintuitive, like replacing wholemeal bread and pasta with white flour options. I could understand why it was imperative to change my diet. I just didn't like it one bit.

The low-salt component of my diet wasn't too difficult, as this was pretty much the way I was eating already. I omitted added salt from my cooking, and prepared my food using fresh ingredients. I stayed away from processed or smoked items; though I must admit I am partial to the occasional bacon sandwich! I understood that a low-salt diet really helps control high blood pressure and helps you to not feel so thirsty. This combination helps to prevent your body from retaining excess fluid. I sure didn't need any more fluid hanging around my ankles, thanks!

7

To drink or not to drink?

I FOUND IT EMOTIONALLY DIFFICULT trying to balance my CKD and my alcohol consumption. I considered my alcohol intake to be fairly low and there were many days in the working week when I didn't drink at all. That part was easy. For me, the most difficult situations occurred on weekends when I would meet up with friends or go out with my boyfriend. I was in my mid-twenties, well-educated and earning my own living. I wanted to enjoy my youth and my freedom!

Eventually, I got very tired of arguing with myself over whether to drink socially with my friends. Having CKD caused me to feel trapped by guilt when I opted to drink and excluded from the social scene when I didn't. I volunteered quite often to be the designated driver, just so I wouldn't have to explain why I wasn't drinking. Sharing the details of my newly diagnosed kidney disease really put a dampener on things, and I hated the pitiful responses and looks I got from those who asked. I had a strict self-imposed rule for Saturday night outings: a *maximum* of three alcoholic drinks!! I knew I would feel guilty the next day if I didn't follow this rule. Not to mention that sitting all evening and drinking over dinner was the worst recipe for gaining two huge pudding-looking feet and 'cankles'.

A few years later I began treating a lovely lady who was a nutritional therapist at a practice in Tonbridge. I consulted her privately and she gave me some great tips regarding acceptable foods and ways to make my diet more varied and interesting. She also evaluated my diet for necessary vitamins and minerals and gave me a list of appropriate dietary supplements. She suggested vodka instead of wine if I did have a tipple when out with my friends – a very good tip indeed!

8
Living with chronic kidney disease

FOR MANY OF THE YEARS BEFORE my transplant, I was reviewed and looked after by the renal team at Guy's and St Thomas' Hospital. I was on medications to control high blood pressure and reduce my high cholesterol. Ramipril, furosemide, amlodipine and atorvastatin were the medications I took for several years. My potassium levels seemed very sensitive to ramipril. Consequently, the dose of this drug was adjusted accordingly from time to time.

I was being seen almost every three to four months and each time I would sign in and head straight for the toilet to do my urine sample, with the same skinny pot the diameter of a two-pence piece and no longer than my finger. I would be hovering above the toilet seat trying to get the urine in the cup and not too much on my hands. It was only after a few years that I noticed some specimen cups that were double the width of the ones I'd been using! How had I never seen these? They reminded me of a see-through version of the cylindrical canisters used to send film off to Kodak for developing. The anticipation of my urinalysis results was a real let-down compared to the excitement of pictures appearing in the post. Then a trot into the room for my 'weigh-in', holding my breath as the numbers settled onto a reading, always hopeful it wouldn't be any higher than the last visit. Finishing with a blood pressure reading, I'd settle in to wait for my consultant to discuss my progress.

I was very lucky that I always had the same consultant, Dr Chowdhury. He was smiley, warm and kind, with his normal clothes always showing beneath an open thigh-length white jacket. There didn't seem to be anything this chap didn't know about the kidneys. He was extremely knowledgeable, open-minded and personable. I had been shown some research regarding taking sodium bicarbonate and its positive effect on kidney function. Dr Chow (as he liked to be called) suggested I take the therapeutic amount to see if it would have any positive effect on my kidneys.

It's hard to know if the sodium bicarbonate had the desired effect, but by 2009 my kidney disease had progressed to stage 4 and my haemoglobin had been steadily falling to around 10gm/dL (the normal level for a woman is 12–15gm/dL). Haemoglobin is what carries oxygen to all the cells of the body.

Even though my kidney function was declining, I felt desperate to pack my life with as many experiences as possible while I still felt well and energetic enough to do so. Throwing caution to the wind, I decided to go travelling!

9
New adventures and a new love

IT WAS AT THIS TIME I DECIDED to go travelling to Australia for three months. I got three months' leave from work and flew to Melbourne. I had a very good friend there named Victoria, who had graduated with me. I travelled on my own and in a small group to Australia's 'Red Centre' to see Uluru (Ayers Rock) and then along the east coast from north to south, eventually getting back down to Melbourne. Vicky and I flew across to New Zealand, and for ten days we travelled around the two islands in a campervan. I even did a skydive on my twenty-eighth birthday! It was just what I needed. I felt alive and challenged and was totally in control of the decisions I made while out there on my own.

There were days I felt alone but knowing I had a loving, supportive family gave me such comfort. Being parted from loved ones really highlights how special they are in our lives. Before leaving for Australia I had started to feel unhappy, though I wasn't quite sure why. I think to some extent I felt I needed to fill my life with more. It was as though my life was on hold, like I was waiting for something and not doing everything I could to go out and fill it with adventure. I got the go-ahead from Dr Chow and took enough medication for the time I was travelling. I was completely out of my comfort zone but felt I was adding to my life experiences and developing some personal strength and confidence. The time I spent travelling solo was great for my self-esteem and quenched my thirst for adventure.

When I returned to England in December 2010, my "fiancé" greeted me late at the airport, his eyes bloodshot and stinking of last night's booze. To say I felt totally deflated would be a massive understatement considering we had been apart for three months. I should have known then that our relationship wasn't going to last. By February of 2011 we had decided to split up. He didn't want to get married and I felt ready to move things along. We were poles apart!

Strangely, the day after we split up, I felt this huge wave of freedom and exhilaration on my drive to work while belting out my rendition of Adele's 'Someone Like You'. That uplifting energy stayed with me into the weekend that followed, and that was when I met Tim, who is now my husband!

The year 2011 was a fantastic year of travelling, adventure and new love! I really grew as a person, with work and all the places I got to see. Tim's attention kept me feeling like an absolute princess. I felt he would always look after me and I loved that, especially with the gradual progression of my kidney disease. This turned out to be the best year I'd had for a long time. I discovered yoga and fell in love with this form of exercise. I taught Pilates, but the hot yoga studio I found in Beckenham was like nothing I had experienced before. I found I was good at it too, which added to my motivation to practise it every other day!

Throughout 2011 my blood pressure remained stable at around 120/80 mmHg. The balance of calcium and phosphate in my blood was constantly monitored and remained stable as well. I increased the sodium bicarbonate supplement as prescribed. If asked, I would have stated that I wasn't experiencing any major signs or symptoms apart from some swelling in my hands and feet if I sat too long and had a glass of wine over dinner.

10

Treating anaemia and low erythropoietin levels

IN 2011 I RECALLED FREQUENT PERIODS of tiredness, especially when driving to work in Tonbridge. It was a forty-five-minute journey, mostly on A roads. I had episodes when I almost fell asleep at the wheel going down the A21 towards Sevenoaks. The last fifteen minutes were difficult, and I struggled to stay awake. The road by and large was quiet, and I would find myself opening the window and putting the radio on loud to avoid falling asleep. I was teaching Pilates classes, often eight per week, and I had moments while teaching when I would feel spaced out, like I wasn't in the room. It's difficult to describe but I just knew it wasn't right. I didn't realise it, but I had become severely anaemic. The management of this condition required erythropoietin therapy and iron infusions. These treatments topped up my stores and improved the level of haemoglobin in my blood.

Receiving an infusion of Venofer, an iron supplement, was an interesting experience. I remember one of the excellent renal nurses at Guy's Hospital administering this via a vein on the inside of my elbow where blood is usually taken. The medication was in a large syringe and looked like treacle, which was very slowly injected into my blood. The strangest part was that after just a few seconds I would get a strange liquorice taste in my mouth while it was being injected. I was warned of this beforehand, but still so startled when I tasted it! I felt so good after this "shot" – energetic and ready to take on anything.

Erythropoietin (EPO) explained...

I hadn't realised that another function of the kidneys is to create a hormone called erythropoietin, or EPO. This hormone is released into the bloodstream by the kidneys when there is a low level of oxygen in the blood. This in turn stimulates the bone marrow to produce red blood cells, which help carry oxygen throughout the body.

When the kidneys are damaged, as mine were, there is less EPO produced and therefore fewer red blood cells produced. With fewer red blood cells, less oxygen is being carried throughout the body. My episodes of altered concentration and tiredness were finally making sense. Luckily, I wasn't suffering with any noticeable shortness of breath or chest pain. Fortunately, at this time I wasn't doing a huge amount of cardiovascular exercise or I might have suffered a heart attack!

I went to see one of the anaemia nurses, who showed me how to self-administer the EPO at home. The medication, called Mircera, came in a kit that included all the necessary sterile components. Hand and skin hygiene was important. There were also clear visual instructions regarding assembling the needle and drug components and how to administer the medication. Luckily, by now, I was comfortable with single-use needles as I used acupuncture regularly in practice alongside my manual therapy. The first couple of times I injected it into my upper thigh, I played around with the location and whether to pucker the skin or keep it flat to see if the sting was any less. There wasn't much difference. The sting was over after a minute or so. By the time I had cleaned up, disposed of the needles in the sharps bin provided and recycled all the paper components, the sting had disappeared. The dose was small, and I self-administered the medication every two weeks.

Mircera required refrigeration and took up the space of a bottle of wine. This wasn't a problem as drinking any wine at this stage was not at the top of my priority list! In fact, I found I wasn't having more than just a glass with a Saturday night meal now as I noticed my hands and feet would swell more quickly. Also, I found I wasn't out with my friends so much, and there was less pressure to keep up with the flow of drinks on a night out. I spent more nights on dates with Tim than anything else, which was wonderful!

11

The parathyroid glands, calcium and phosphate

I HAD DEVELOPED HYPERPARATHYROIDISM at this point, with a PTH of 220ng/L (normal levels range between 10 and 65ng/L). This was yet another revelation regarding the function of the kidneys! How could one organ do so many things?

The balance, or 'homeostasis', of calcium, phosphate and vitamin D levels are all influenced by the function of the kidneys and have a secondary effect on the parathyroid glands. These glands are in the front of your neck, beneath the thyroid gland. There is a complex relationship between the kidneys, parathyroid glands, bones and intestines. The parathyroid glands monitor and control calcium in the body. When the kidneys are damaged, they reduce the filtering of phosphates out of the body, so it accumulates. This disorder, called hyperphosphataemia, causes the parathyroid to increase its hormone production.

The kidney also regulates the amount of calcium in the blood and bones. When the kidneys are diseased the amount of calcium being released is reduced, which stimulates the parathyroid to increase production of its hormone. This causes calcium to move out of the bones and into the blood, which in turn can potentially reduce bone strength and have a negative impact on the cardiovascular (heart) system. So I was now prescribed the medication alfacalcidol.

My phosphate level was also elevated, and my dietician suggested a low phosphate diet (alongside the low sodium and potassium) to help bring this down to the acceptable range. I was not too thrilled about this as I'm sure you can imagine! The list of banned foods just kept getting longer and longer... Suggested changes included severely limiting or full avoidance of dairy products. This meant no milk, ice cream or cheese. I love cheese! There were other things like avoiding beans and lentils; however, I didn't tend to eat a huge amount of these anyway. The private nutritionist I had consulted, Amanda Reuter at Better Health – Naturally Ltd, suggested some alternatives like oat or soy milk and dairy-free cream cheese, so I had a few options at least.

12

Physical exercise and stage 4 CKD

I REALLY ENJOYED HOT YOGA CLASSES, but I think the elevated environmental temperature was detrimental to my kidney function and to my overall health. The temperature would often be around forty-two degrees in the studio. Although it helped my flexibility getting into poses, I was left very tired afterwards. After discussion with my renal consultant, I decided to return to a traditional yoga studio, where a normal room temperature would be maintained.

Tim and I had also been doing some long bike rides in hopes of doing a cycling challenge from London to Paris. It was a personal challenge Tim and his father, Richard, had set before he passed away earlier that year from colon cancer. Tim and his father had completed a London to Land's End cycle challenge just the year before! Tim's dad completed this challenge with a colostomy bag and I was so inspired by his fortitude and determination!

I did a few long cycles and even managed twenty miles a few months before my transplant. I could manage them but felt incredibly tired afterwards and found that my hands and face would become tight like they were swollen. I had a feeling challenging myself to over two hundred miles in three days was not within my grasp at this point. My kidney function just wasn't up to it.

By the end of 2011 I was transferred to the advanced kidney care clinic. My kidney function had continued to deteriorate, and this move signalled the start of preparations for my transplant as well as discussions about haemodialysis.

Part Two

Transplant Preparations

13
Transplant surgery and dialysis talks

DURING MY FIRST APPOINTMENT AT THE advanced kidney care unit, my renal consultant and I began the conversation about renal transplantation and dialysis. This came as no surprise considering the deterioration of my kidney function. He explained that there are two pathways of donation: I would have either a living donor or a deceased one. He also gave me some information about attending the transplant education sessions. I was hopeful for a pre-emptive transplant from a family member who was willing to donate; the prospect of dialysis seemed so dismal. Dialysis was time-consuming and would limit my availability to see my own osteopathy patients. A fistula would need to be surgically implanted in my arm, which made me feel really squeamish. If I could receive a transplant before requiring dialysis, I would be a very lucky and grateful lady.

I started having chats with my parents and my brother, Dean, regarding my kidney function. Dean came forward immediately and said he would be happy to be tested as a possible donor. He's two years older and lived in North London with his girlfriend. He worked full time and exercised lots, playing football and going to the gym. He wasn't a smoker and he drank alcohol just socially on the weekends. He was a very good candidate.

I felt so relieved that he had suggested it. This was a huge relief, as there are so many people waiting for a transplant who have no one, family or otherwise, who could donate. He volunteered to attend the informational meetings with me. I really felt like I needed another pair of ears to listen to all the information that was flooding in now regarding transplantation and other options such as dialysis.

I was given a DVD and booklet titled *Your Kidneys, Your Choice* and another booklet, *Gift of Life*, to read prior to my next consultation. Details of my medical history and current health information were forwarded to the living donor team. They would contact Dean.

My hepatitis B immunity levels were checked, as I had received this vaccine a few months before the onset of symptoms of renal disease and they wanted to determine if I needed a booster.

By this stage, I was also prescribed sodium bicarbonate, 1.5g twice daily, and my ramipril dose was reduced to 2.5mg once daily. My creatinine level was 293umol/L and my eGFR was 16ml/min.

When will I need my transplant and how long will it last?

In January of 2012 Dean attended my appointment in the advanced kidney care clinic with me. The question I often asked the consultants was "When will I need a transplant?" At this appointment the consultant was unsure and replied that it really depended on the rate of change in my kidney function. It was a little bit like a dangling carrot at this point. After reading all the information regarding transplantation, it seemed that this was the best treatment option possible, an opportunity for a new lease on life! I could go back to a regular diet with no restrictions, be able to exercise at an intensity that I would like to and potentially start a family. I could really see a future with Tim and the feeling seemed mutual. Tim has his own physiotherapy business and was really supportive with my health issues.

It was explained to me that the length of time the transplanted kidney will last is variable, and in some cases of FSGS, the disease can reoccur in the transplanted kidney, thereby reducing the life span of the donated organ. This was a chance I was willing to take, and Dean was in complete agreement. We received the good news that Dean was a suitable candidate. He was contacted by the recipient transplant coordinator to begin his donor assessment.

What happens during transplant surgery?

Honestly, I didn't try to absorb much of the information I received about the intricacies of the actual transplant surgery. I just knew this was my best chance of leading a normal life again, so any risks or gory details seemed insignificant in the scheme of things. However, for informational purposes of this book, I felt it was necessary to give the reader a good basic explanation of the surgery.

Basically, the wonderful, amazing, super selfless donor is taken into the operating theatre first for the talented surgeon to harvest one of their kidneys (usually the best or largest one of the two), along with the attached ureter. The ureter is the tube that carries urine from the kidney to the bladder. The vital signs of the donor are monitored very closely during the procedure; the incision is closed, and the donor is taken to recovery for careful observation.

Meanwhile, the very grateful and excited recipient (me) is taken to theatre and an incision is made in the lower abdomen where the donated kidney will be situated. The recipient's poorly functioning kidneys are left in place unless they are causing issues such as pain or infection.

Then the kidney is 'plumbed in'. The recipient's blood vessels are attached to the donor kidney's blood vessels, and finally the ureter is attached to the recipient's bladder.

A small plastic tube called a stent is often inserted into the ureter to help keep it open and facilitate the flow of urine into the bladder. This gets taken out later, usually six to twelve weeks after surgery. The surgeries for donor and recipient each take around three hours to complete.

The dialysis back-up plan

My renal consultant and I discussed haemodialysis as part of my transplant preparations. I had done a lot of reading about the subject and understood that dialysis must be considered as a back-up plan in case there were any unforeseen delays with my transplant. As I've mentioned previously, I wasn't thrilled with the prospect of having a fistula inserted into my arm or about the huge amount of time that would be spent in dialysis every week. I had decided that if I needed short-term dialysis, I'd have it done at an in-centre unit. It's nice that dialysis has progressed so much and that patients can be dialysed at home now.

14

Miscarriage

MY PERIODS WERE VERY SPORADIC and irregular by this stage of my kidney disease. I really felt that my risk of getting pregnant at this point was very low. Tim and I decided to use a barrier method of contraception, opting for condoms. We both felt I was on so much medication that the contraceptive pill didn't seem a very wise choice. Also, my blood pressure became elevated in my late teens when I was put on a contraceptive pill, which was prescribed to treat my acne as well. I didn't want anything to cause an increase in my blood pressure.

In May of 2012 I had a miscarriage, which I was very taken aback by, as I didn't realise I had been pregnant. On reflection, I think I may have been about four weeks late for one of my periods and then I had an extremely heavy bleed. I didn't know it was possible to bleed that much during a period. It did occur to me that this may have been because I didn't have a period the previous month. After a few days, the bleeding subsided somewhat and was more like my usual monthly flow.

I was treating patients in Tonbridge when I got an almighty stomach cramp and began bleeding heavily once more. At this stage I thought this was very unlike any period I had had in the past. My colleague at work suggested that I may have been having a miscarriage.

After another couple of days it eased slightly again, and I went to see my local GP about it. He did not seem to be worried and said that it may have been due to a missed period. A day or two later, this awful wave of pain came on again. Travelling home, I had the worst pain I had ever experienced. Blood was flooding my seat; I knew something was seriously wrong. I managed to pull over into the car park at a restaurant in Farnborough, Kent. I'm not sure if I did it intentionally, but where I pulled over was directly opposite the local hospital. I was in so much pain and was bleeding so heavily that I was almost delirious by now.

I called Tim and told him where I was and what was happening. I couldn't bear to sit in the car, so I grabbed a Pilates mat out of my boot, laid it out on the ground next to the car, and curled up in a ball on it until Tim and his sister, a qualified A&E nurse, came to help me. I'm not sure of any of the details after that. They got me into a wheelchair and to the hospital where I was seen immediately. Tim's sister, Nikki, took charge of the situation. I was bleeding very heavily and was worried that I may need a blood transfusion. I recalled some information from the transplant education meetings that said to avoid unnecessary blood transfusions. Exposure to multiple blood donations may cause an immune response and increase the chance of rejection of the donor kidney. I didn't want anything ruining my chance of a successful transplant as it was getting near to the time of my surgery. Thankfully, they honoured my request. The team at the Princess Royal University Hospital were outstanding. They diagnosed that I was indeed having a miscarriage and would need a dilation and curettage (D&C) to remove any remaining cells that were retained in my body.

While recovering at home I felt so teary and emotionally upset for quite a while after this. I think it was more from the shock of everything that had happened, replaying the situation over in my head and thinking about all the what-ifs. I think the change in hormones contributed too. I was so grateful that I didn't get a blood transfusion. The medics requested that I take time to recover fully as I really was on the cusp of needing one. I cannot say I felt any sense of loss in my situation as I didn't realise I had been pregnant, and therefore hadn't started to look forward to the possibility of having a baby.

At the first renal check-up I had following this event, I was given information about the renal psychology support system and information that discussed the importance of reliable contraception. I did reflect on how careless I had been to not be more diligent with contraception. This was a really important stage for me and the situation could have ended disastrously in so many ways. I needed to be as fit for transplant surgery as possible, even as my kidney function continued to deteriorate.

15

Work-up for transplant

BOTH MUM AND DAD HAD BEEN assessed as possible donors. Dad was fifty-nine and Mum was fifty-eight. Both were in good health, a little on the podgy side but non-smokers who consumed alcohol only rarely. Dad was very disappointed to find out that his blood pressure wasn't good enough and his weight too high to be considered as a donor, although it did spur him on to lose some weight and get more active. His blood pressure improved too. Mum, however, was an excellent candidate, and she had some great blood test results. How lucky was I? I now had a choice of two donors: my mother and my brother.

My work-up involved having a Doppler scan of my veins, especially in the lower abdomen, a chest X-ray and an ECG. Thankfully, all came back clear. I was also required to have a dental review. This was to assess the health of my teeth and gums prior to surgery. Following surgery, I would be on immunosuppressant medication, which would increase the likelihood of developing infections more easily. I was also seen by a consultant surgeon for a transplant assessment. My eGFR at this stage was 12mL/min, with my haemoglobin at 8.8g/dL.

It was at this appointment that we had discussions about whether my brother or my mother would be my donor. I felt so fortunate to be "deciding" which kidney to use. For many, it is a long, anxious wait for a deceased donor to become available and be a match! It was thought that my brother's kidney may have been marginally better as he was younger, but we also had to consider that I was only twenty-nine years old and may need another kidney at some point in my life. The team suggested I take my mother's healthy kidney now, with the possibility of using Dean's kidney as a back-up should I need another transplant in the future. I felt so lucky I had two to choose from. I did feel a sense of guilt that someone I love very much had to have an operation for me. But I had complete faith in the medical team. I kept reflecting on the information that suggested there is a very high success rate from a living kidney donation and very low risk of death.

It was still such a huge, selfless act from my mother. One day I asked her if she was sure about her decision to donate and I will never forget her reply. She simply said, "I brought you into this world, and I will do all I can to keep you in this world!"

The statement brings me to tears even thinking about it now, the selfless act of a mother for her child. I was extremely lucky her kidneys were healthy, and she was fit enough to undergo an operation of this magnitude and complexity.

I will be forever in her debt.

16

Three months before transplant

MY KIDNEY FUNCTION CONTINUED to deteriorate. My creatinine level was 431umol/L and my eGFR was 11mL/min. I didn't feel too unwell at all and continued working three to four days a week. I would feel tired after work or after doing vigorous exercise. My face was rather puffy and I had gained a little weight.

We managed to get on a family holiday to Lindos on the Greek island of Rhodes. I remember feeling well and enjoyed the restful days of sunbathing and eating out. I often felt as the day went on that I would look a little bit larger around my waist and my ankles would get puffy much more quickly when sitting down at dinner. There was a sense of tightness in my feet and if I wore strappy shoes or a court shoe, my puffy feet would get imprints in them from my shoe. The imprints would wear off by the morning.

The hospital wanted to see me on a regular basis – every seven to ten days to monitor my bloods. They also spoke about the possibility of needing a brief period of dialysis before the transplant if the operation was not imminent and said it may be sensible to go ahead with inserting the fistula. I did not like the sound of that! This gave me more anxiety than the operation. If I needed dialysis, I would have to face my fears about the dreaded fistula that made me feel faint just from the thought of it. Getting light-headed during blood tests was always something I had had an issue with, and by now I had undergone a fair few.

While at university I'd set myself a challenge to be able to donate a full pint of blood. It took three attempts as during the previous two I had become so faint they discontinued the process. Oh, the pride I felt when they finally took a whole pint!! It was immense!

I was more than ready to go ahead with the surgery by this point.

17
The ReMIND research study

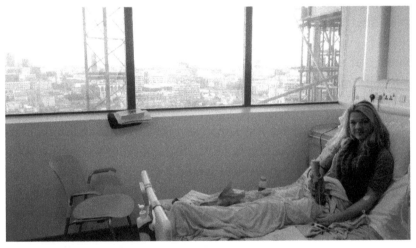

12 October 2012.
At Guy's Hospital having Rituximab administered via an intravenous drip
for the ReMIND research study.

I WAS ASKED BY THE GUY'S AND St Thomas' research team if I would take part in a study as a renal patient. The title was 'A Randomised Trial of Rituximab in Induction Therapy for Living Donor Renal Transplantation', abbreviated to *ReMIND* (thankfully).

They wanted to see if taking a single dose of the drug Rituximab would allow a reduced dosage of other anti-rejection drugs.

The side effects of these drugs can cause damage to the donor kidney. This drug had been shown to reduce rejection in one study and was being used regularly for transplants with a high risk of rejection. The drug targets B cells and destroys some of them, thereby reducing transplant rejection.

If I were to receive this drug prior to surgery, the positive outcome certainly outweighed the risk of side effects. If chosen, I would receive the drug two weeks before transplant and then receive the anti-rejection medications given, as per protocol, but would receive only one week of steroids, rather than having to take them continuously...This seemed to be a much better option. I already knew the consequences of long-term steroid use: increased chance of osteoporosis, diabetes, weight gain, to name just a few. I had all my fingers and toes crossed I would be included in the study. And I was!

On 12 October I had Rituximab administered via an intravenous drip, which took a few hours. I felt a little nervous as it was a stark reminder that in a few weeks I would be back in hospital, putting on the same blue-checked cotton hospital gown in readiness for major surgery. I understood that being part of the study required some extra blood samples that would be taken at the same time as the routine post-transplant ones. To be honest, I was really grateful and happy to give them my blood for this study. It was such a small ask for such a big gain.

Dear Diary,

12 October 2012, Rituximab - 18 days pre-transplant

I was so pleased when Tim said he was coming with me today. He cancelled his morning of patients just to support me! He set off early, running for the train only to then miss it coming in at New Beckenham Station...doh! It's not the first time. I think that's the problem with living so close to the station...You leave the house too late. Anyway, the next train was ten minutes after. I knew I was going to be late, but I usually wait for appointments at the hospital, so I didn't panic too much. I got a call from Jay, the head researcher of the ReMIND study, making sure I was on my way in. I suddenly realised how important my presence was going to be today, as well as the reality and significance of the unusual situation of the event.

After taking some bloods, Jay took them personally to the research lab and took us up to the fifteenth floor, which was the research unit. It was very bright and exceptionally clean, with amazing views of London. I felt important and cared for, with offerings of tea or coffee while I answered questionnaires on the computer. Jay had two other researchers following him, learning about the study and the format of each part.

Guy's Hospital is funding an investigational drug study trial on Rituximab, and only sixteen others have received it within the study so far. I felt so fortunate to be included.

We had a chance to have a drink and snack up on the sixteenth floor, which was technically for staff members only. However, once again, this seemed to be a little VIP treatment offered to us today. I sat with Tim for about forty-five minutes looking across London, absorbing the views of St Paul's and the London Eye. The day was *bright and sunny with a dusting of clouds that made London look so vibrant and colourful.*

We headed back down to the fifteenth floor and were shown to a room with two beds, a big plasma screen TV and yet another wonderful view of London from the window. It was rather chilly, so I kept my coat on initially. I took the opportunity to lie on the bed while waiting for the results from my bloods. I felt strange at first, lying on the bed...My instinct was that you only lie on hospital beds when you're feeling very poorly – which I did not.

At about 1.30pm I was given a dose of paracetamol along with one steroid injection and one injection of antihistamine, which made me drowsy. Thank goodness I had eaten some lunch Tim got for us just prior to this because I could barely keep my eyes open. At 2pm the infusion of Rituximab started at a very slow drip rate, which was gradually increased. I was so grateful to have Tim beside me. He was the supportive presence I needed but I did not feel any burden of having to keep him amused. He continued working away on the laptop, doing his "admin" that he is always so motivated with. The infusion finished at 4.45pm.

I made my way home on the train, still feeling very drowsy and a little paranoid about whether anyone on the carriage was sniffling or coughing with a cold. Rituximab is a monoclonal antibody and can make you more susceptible to serious infections. I was advised to avoid anyone with a cold as much as possible. Very difficult on public transport!

After having a sleep when I got home, I reflected on my day and felt I should write this experience down. There may come a time in the future when I'll want to return to my writings for reference. Today has been a significant day in my life, and so I have written about it.

18

A surgery date and Mum's final work-up

THE DATE OF THE SURGERY WAS BOOKED for 30 October 2012. My blood pressure remained well-controlled at 130/88. The consultant described me as having no signs of fluid overload. My eGFR was now 7ml/min. I was taken off ramipril due to having too much potassium in my blood. By mid-October it was looking like my living donor transplant would be classed as pre-emptive, in that I would not require dialysis. I felt so blessed; it was unbelievable. Everything seemed to be falling into place.

Mum had quite a few blood tests and became quite fond of the lady who was organising her work-up for the operation, the independent living donor advocate (ILDA). I really didn't get to know this lady or that team and, looking back, I think this is to reduce the chance of any conflicts of interest. The team began with taking a medical screening, asking questions about Mum's medical health, followed by a blood test to see if she would be compatible with me.

Lots of information was relayed regarding possible risks and benefits of donation, along with emotional aspects: family, health and future employment. It was all kept completely confidential. There were more in-depth questions regarding psychological evaluation, making sure there was no pressure from friends or family or promise of a monetary incentive. They made sure Mum was in good mental health. The extensive medical tests also included a chest X-ray and ECG to check for heart or lung disease. Radiological testing was performed on her two kidneys, looking at the blood vessels. Urine testing, gynaecological examination and cancer screening were all done, along with the compatibility blood sample tests. The blood tests also check for things such as hepatitis and glucose intolerance as well as kidney function.

Mum seemed happy to do these, and Dad would go along too. I think she also often felt like a VIP, especially when she was recognised by the living donor evaluation team. As well she should! She was doing an awesome thing.

19
Diary extracts twelve days pre-transplant

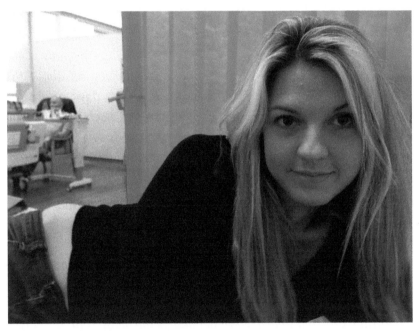

29 October 2012, Admission Day.
Feeling uneasy about lying on the ward bed when I wasn't feeling sick.

Dear Diary,

18 October 2012 - 12 days before transplant

Gosh, what a day. Mum and I met at London Bridge, and I immediately felt a wave of guilt sweep over me when I saw Mummy looking a little sleepy and disgruntled that she had commuted on a busy train in rush hour. Holding her arm, I tried to make up for it with some warm cuddles and chatter. We were quickly taken in for our bloods to be tested. We jokingly call the phlebotomists in the kidney clinic 'vampires' even though they are all really lovely and bubbly. Jay (the research lead for the ReMIND study) was there at the clinic, ready for his ten small tubes to be filled with blood for the drug study.

Mum's transplant coordinator, Miri, with her huge friendly smile, whisked us off for some swab testing, and information about the immunosuppressant drug I will need to take two days before the operation. Then there was a trip to have a repeat electrocardiogram (ECG) for both of us and a chest X-ray for me. It amazes me how quickly these tests are performed when requested by the renal team. I never seem to have to wait long. It is such an efficient service.

After a quick tea stop, we headed back for an education session. In attendance were two hopeful kidney recipients and another kidney donor. One of the recipients had already had a kidney lasting twenty years and was due to have a second donated by his daughter. The talk was packed with information about what items to take to the hospital, and what to expect the day before and on the day of the operation. I started to feel overwhelmed by the detail that was given, especially about the surgical procedures. I became reflective on the fact Mummy had to go through this. I kept thinking...Bloody hell, this is really happening, isn't it?!

I was shocked to see the number of pills I will need to take post-operatively. It really highlighted how this really isn't a cure as such, but the best chance I had for surviving. We filled in questionnaires for a PhD study that looked at emotional implications of kidney disease and the impact it has had on our lives. It was an eye-opener to just how fortunate I am to be having the pre-emptive live donor transplant surgery that Guy's Hospital is arranging for me. I am still working two days a week and feeling relatively well in that I do not feel nauseated and still have my appetite. I think the most important thing is that I have not had to go on dialysis while waiting for this transplant to happen. I am such a lucky girl! It's made me look at my body in a totally different light. I remember having a conversation with my ex-boyfriend when I was newly diagnosed. I recalled saying that I likened myself to a weak runt of a litter and if it was down to survival of the fittest, I would have been eaten up by now! Now I believe my body IS strong and even though my eGFR is only 7 (normal is 70–100), I continue to remain active and to work and feel relatively well! My body's ability to deal with this disease has amazed me.

So, our last stop was back up to the fifteenth floor to the research clinic to see Jay once more before the day of surgery. He asked about whether I was willing to have a bone marrow biopsy as part of a separate research project on B cells. My first thought was to talk it out with Tim! There was no pressure for an answer today so I will let him know.

We headed home and I felt relieved I had rescheduled my afternoon of patients and two Pilates classes in the evening. It had been an emotional and information-packed day. I just appreciated the evening to reflect on some of what was said and to enjoy a dinner with Tim and his mum who have been amazingly supportive through the entire ordeal. I am so blessed to have both in my life.

Dear Diary,

27 October 2012 – last day at work, 3 days before transplant

My last morning was full with patients, all lovely and wishing me well. I have been overwhelmed by the number of cards, presents and kind messages I have received throughout the week. Some particularly significant gestures have been a dinner arranged and paid for by my Tonbridge clinic work colleagues, flowers and vouchers from some of my Pilates clients and some fabulous gifts from family including Lisa [my auntie] and Nikki. I got emotional at the work meal three days ago when saying goodbye to everyone. I was so touched at the effort made by so many colleagues. My body was showing signs of nerves building about the operation as I couldn't seem to shake off a stomach ache that began in the afternoon and continued into the evening. It lasted a good couple of days and got worse every time I ate. At first, I thought it was something completely life threatening like a stomach ulcer. After a level-headed conversation with my therapist friends at work I realised it was probably nerves combined with a touch of constipation. Their suggestion was to just have a strong coffee to get the bowels moving. It worked! Maybe the therapeutic talking therapy with those wise ladies was a catalyst too.

I felt pretty distracted the rest of Saturday and Sunday when spending time with Tim and having dinner at my parents'. Mum seems very calm and level-headed about it all, concerned about what to pack more than anything. Maybe this is her coping strategy. She will arrive on the morning of the operation, which I hope will allow her to have a good night's sleep at home. I managed to keep distracted with my newly delivered iPhone 5. I needed to set it up this weekend too, and just in the nick of time.

Dear Diary,

29 October 2012 - 1 day before transplant, Admission Day

After a nice reassuring cuddle with Tim this morning, I got up and started packing. Strangely, it felt like I was packing for a trip or holiday, only instead of taking a variety of bikinis, it was a variety of pyjamas. I have been inundated with messages throughout the day, really kind 'thinking of you' texts and Facebook messages.

Mum and Dad came over in the morning for a cup of tea, which was lovely. Lisa [my mum's youngest sister and amazingly supportive aunt] arrived to stay and support my parents during this period of time. I showed them all my cards and gifts and commented to Lisa that it feels like my birthday has come early with all the attention and gifts. I think the gift I'm about to receive from Mum is the best early birthday present I could ever hope to receive.

Tim and I set off on the train and got to the kidney clinic in Guy's for my 2pm appointment. Jay was there and showed me through to the 'vampires' for another twenty tubes of blood to be taken, again. He showed us up to the Richard Bright ward on the sixth floor. It was warm and a little stuffy, as wards tend to be, with plenty of space between the beds. There were quite a few visitors, but no one was overly noisy.

I sat on the bed, which was made up for me once I arrived, number twenty-three. Mum will be in bed twenty-four tomorrow. I felt a wave of relief that we were allowed to leave the hospital to get a bite to eat once I'd seen the doctor, which didn't happen until 6pm! It felt odd to be there, as I looked and felt so well compared to those lying in other bays. I just kept thinking that while I may look like a fraud, my bloods and my kidney function were poor and told a different story. I just kept telling myself how lucky I was to be here at this stage.

A doctor put an intravenous cannula in my hand, then Tim and I went for supper just outside Guy's at the London Bridge Hotel Bar and Lounge. We called it my 'last supper', before I needed to be nil by mouth and before hospital food would be my dining option for the next few days. We heartily ate a platter of mini burgers and chunky chips that were absolutely delicious.

We got back to the ward and I felt ready to change into my pyjamas and get ready for bed. The evening nurse seems very sweet and caring. Tim has contact information for all of my friends and family and will send emails to keep everyone updated. He has been by my side all afternoon, just getting on with his admin work and being such a comforting presence.

Part Three

Transplant Surgery

20
Transplant Day diary extract

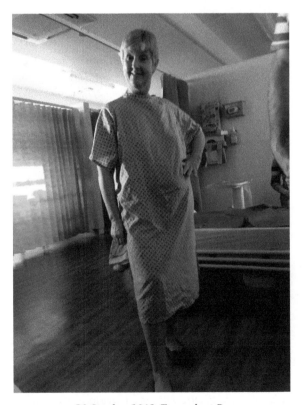

30 October 2012, Transplant Day.
Mummy showing her wonderful sense of humour to lighten the
apprehension we were all feeling.

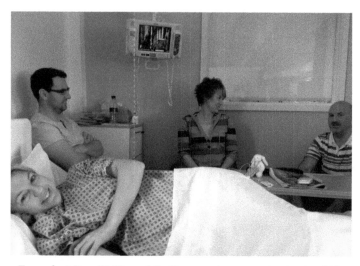

Transplant Day. Waiting while Mum was in surgery having her kidney removed. My brother sits behind me (left), Auntie Lisa in the middle and Dad is sitting on the right. Tim is taking the photograph.

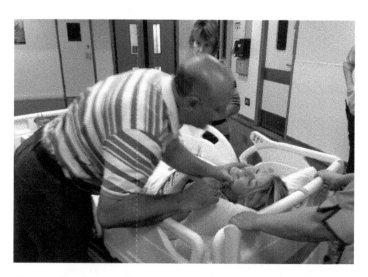

Getting taken down to theatre, putting a brave face on for my Dad, who is squeezing my cheeks – one of his endearing expressions of love and affection. I was full of adrenaline and shaky.

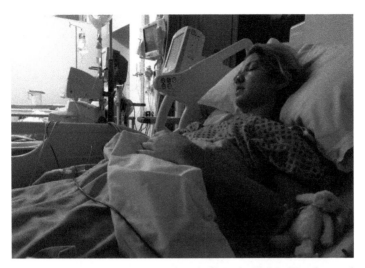

A few hours following surgery, asleep back in the Richard Bright ward at Guy's Hospital. Mum is asleep in the bed next to me.

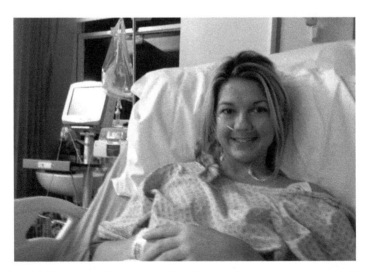

Day 1 following my kidney transplant. I was feeling sore but very grateful.

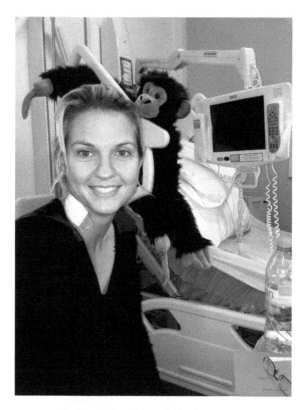

Discharge Day, 5 days following surgery.

Dear Diary,

30 October 2012 - Day of Transplant (written a week later)

The day started early with Mum, Dad, Dean and Auntie Lisa arriving around 7am. Mum was shown to her bed next to mine and given her lovely hospital-issued gown and support socks. The atmosphere was light-hearted, but I was feeling nervous. We laughed at Mum posing for a picture in the blue-and-white checked hospital gown and slippers, looking like she owned it. This was all good to keep the mood a little less tense and worried. They took Mum off around 8.25am and we had a little kiss and cuddle before she left. No tears, we just tried to stay very positive and upbeat. Dad got quite emotional when he said goodbye to Mum before she headed down in the lift. I could see he tried to compose himself before coming back to sit next to my bed.

While Mum was in theatre, I remained in bed with a plasma drip attached to me to keep me super hydrated. I had the odd wave of nerves, thinking it will not be long until I'm taken off. I don't think you can ever fully prepare yourself for what is about to happen, but I just tried to remain positive. I knew that this was the only possible means to a way of improving my life. Besides, Mum has already done the most selfless thing one could ever be asked to do in donating one of her healthy kidneys.

An Irish girl around my age was in the bed opposite mine and had received a donated kidney just five days previously. She was sitting up eating breakfast and appeared to be comfortable. This was a promising sight. Hopefully I will look that well in five days' time!

I had a caring, gentle nurse help me get into my robe and socks after having a brief wash and taking anti-rejection tablets in preparation for surgery. We got the call around 12.30pm that the donor kidney retrieval was nearly complete, and I was about to be taken down. I really tried to hold it together, as I got a massive wave of emotion and panic. This was it! This was the moment we had spoken about for such a long time and it was happening now! Swallowing back a couple of tears so I didn't set Dad off, I put on a brave face, smiled and laughed and said, "Finally, I'm off for a few hours' solid sleep!" Tim, Dad and Lisa walked with the bed to the lift. Once in the lift, we came out just outside the theatre room in the anaesthesia preparatory area. It was cold, or at least I felt very cold and shivery. After a few questions from a male and a female anaesthetist, the man put a mask over my mouth and gave me an injection in my IV cannula. I knew that was it! I was going under and the room faded out after becoming slightly brighter in colour.

The first person I saw in recovery was the same male anaesthetist. I grabbed his hand and thanked him straight away. I felt emotional and wanted to cry, maybe from relief that it was done but also that I was awake again. Everyone helping in the recovery room was so gentle and kind. The female nurse reminded me of Myleene Klass, very pretty and she had a very gentle nature. I could hear other nurses trying to wake up a patient lying in a bed adjacent to mine..."Trevor, do you know where you are?" was repeated more times than I could count...I was instructed to keep pressing a button to dispense pain relief to me while I was there. Apparently I had been there since 5pm and it was now around 8pm. Once the changeover of nurses had happened on the ward, I was wheeled back up. I couldn't wait to see all my loved ones. It was like a little fan base, all waiting by my bed just as I had left them. Mum was lying in her bed asleep and I felt incredibly drowsy. I couldn't really keep my eyes open but just had enough in me to joke about giving autographs to my fans in the morning. I was in pain but so sleepy. Everyone kissed me goodnight and I fell asleep.

21

Our hospital recovery

Dear Diary,

Day 1 post-transplant
31 October 2012

MY FIRST NIGHT IS A LITTLE BLURRY. I was awakened frequently throughout the night for bloods to be taken and medication to be given. There was a different patient in the bed opposite mine, as the Irish girl had gone home! This patient had a persistent and very irritating cough, which didn't help with my restless night. I was shown how to use the button for the patient-controlled analgesia (PCA) pump. It contained opioid pain medicine such as morphine and helped dampen the pain. The curtain was pulled between Mum and me and I felt frustrated that I couldn't see her. Once the doctor had been round, I called out to Mum.

"Are you awake, Mum?" I said through the curtain.

"Why have they pulled the curtain across?" Mum replied sounding disgruntled. I felt reassured that she wasn't doing too badly, as she

was already expressing her opinion about our space being divided. Mum asked the ward nurse as she passed by if the curtain could be pulled back and we turned heads to look at each other.

"Hello," I said in a cheery voice, fairly softly as my tummy felt sore just speaking.

"Hello, Daughter," Mum replied, sounding weary but with that familiar comforting tone that was happy to hear from me.

I felt relieved that Mum was awake, and we could see and speak to each other. We were able to keep the curtain open unless one of the doctors or nurses was coming to discuss test results or perform a procedure such as wound dressing checks. We both liked it this way; it felt like our space to rehabilitate together, to keep each other company. We were in this together. If the curtain did happen to be left closed, it was no more than five minutes before we managed to get it reopened again by the helpful nurses on the ward.

We were both incredibly uncomfortable with abdominal pain and were constantly pressing our PCA buttons, Mum slightly more often than me. I think she made herself feel sick from taking too much. Tim arrived first, around 11am, and watched me struggle to eat a mouthful of mashed potato and fromage frais. I was a little nauseated, but fortunately held down my medications. I managed to sit quite upright in the bed and was given some great news about my kidney function when the doctors came around. My creatinine level had gone down from 690 to 320 in just sixteen hours and my eGFR had increased from 6 to 23! Apparently, the kidney started working as soon as it was 'plumbed in' and before the ureter had even been attached to the bladder! So they had to act fast. The doctors were very pleased with the results so far and so was I. I could not have asked for anything better. My new kidney was working straight away.

I continued to feel better as the day progressed, but Mum continued to feel poorly. She was very uncomfortable and nauseated. I felt so sorry for her and guilty because she had done this wonderful thing for me and now she was the one who felt sick. Her symptoms did improve by the evening and eventually she managed to eat some dinner.

Lisa, my incredibly caring and supportive Auntie helped me to wash as I was feeling so smelly. Having a urinary catheter is uncomfortable and my personal hygiene felt below par. I felt human once more after having a simple body wash. Lisa has had a nurturing role in my life since I was born, looking after my brother and me in the school holidays, taking us out for day trips. So often she would spoil us with gifts, and always expressed lots of affection and love. She is my mum's youngest sister, with an age gap of thirteen years, and has such a kind and comforting character. I liken her to our personal angel sent from God. Lisa has been the best nurse we could have ever had, and happy to help in any way. With her, I have no shyness about getting undressed or tending to personal care. Thank goodness she was able to stay and help at this critical time for both of us.

Tim managed to get to stay until 10.15pm. He has been so supportive too, not only to me but also to Mum, helping her get comfortable in bed. We drifted off to sleep, not waking until 5am... this time by a different noisy patient!

Dear Diary,

Day 2 post-transplant
1 November 2012

The very annoying noisy patient managed to wake the whole ward around 5am, moaning about how much pain she was in, even though she was more than capable of getting out of her bed, downstairs and outside to have a bloody cigarette!

The nurse who took over this morning had a slower pace, and I couldn't wait for Lisa to arrive – our very own Florence Nightingale, the best nurse we could have wished for.

It took a while for the doctors to do their rounds, but again they seemed very happy with our progress. The surgeon, Dr Nicos Kessaris, also popped by to see me and I shook his hand and thanked him for his wonderful work. I was like a bumbling teenager who had just seen her pop idol, although I'm sure the profession of a surgeon is far more impactful than that of a pop prince. He reiterated what was said previously about the kidney working on the operating table. This seems to not always be the case with kidney transplants, and I felt so grateful, both for that and to him for his skilled hands.

I was feeling so smelly; it was really starting to bother me. As soon as the doctors left the ward, I asked our nurse to help me up in order to wash myself. Mum's catheter was taken out, which was pleasing but she was unable to get comfortable in her chair that sat next to the bed.

I was determined to get up and wash but did a pretty poor job on my own. Still smelling of things one shouldn't smell like, I prayed my wonderful aunt would be arriving soon. I continued to stay sitting in the chair so Dad would be able to see my improvement. Sure enough, when both Lisa and Dad arrived, they were very surprised and pleased to see us up. Tim arrived at the same time too. Lisa and Dad helped Mum to the toilet to give her a wash and then got her as comfortable as possible in the chair next to me.

I felt I needed the same. Lisa helped and I managed to have a thorough wash and do a few very small rabbit-like droppings in the toilet. Opioid pain medication really can cause constipation. I felt so undignified but thank goodness Lisa had been at the hospital to help us. She has been the tonic and amazing female support that we have both needed.

We had Tim's mum pop in to see us before they went off for some dinner, and a surprise visit from a cousin on my dad's side of the family. It was sweet of her to visit, but by then I felt exhausted. At one stage we had five visitors beside our beds.

I don't think we could have asked for a better second day with what we have managed to achieve. I hope tomorrow continues in the same way.

Dear Diary,

Day 3 post-transplant...a day of laughter and incontinence!
2 November 2012

I was awakened during the night by concerned nurses as my blood pressure was elevated. A nice doctor encouraged me to use the PCA as it would help control my pain, which would in turn decrease my blood *pressure. I slept well after that but woke feeling a little drowsy. It was 6am, and they were getting blood from my central intravenous line and having me sit on chair scales to get my weight.*

Mum got rid of all her wires and managed a few independent trips to the loo. However, she strained her abdominal muscles and incision getting into bed, which made her sore. Her breathing was a little shallow, so the doctors suggested a chest X-ray to check her lungs. The X-ray came back clear, but they reinforced she needed to be upright in the chair and do some deep breathing exercises to expand her lungs, which she did.

My drain was removed from my abdomen, which made me feel a little woozy. I remember having to take a breath in while it was taken out, which probably helped with the discomfort, but it was an odd sensation. The dressing on my incision was attached to the few remaining pubic hairs I had left after my pre-op shave. That was very uncomfortable coming off. I guess I didn't need those hairs anyway.

Mum and I were up and in our chairs early and had eaten our lunch together by the time Dad and Lisa arrived. Mum had already wet herself from laughing, and both of us had sore abdomens from the laughter. Lots of things were setting us off today: things said in patients' conversations with visitors, unusual patient voices and later the recollection of Mum wetting herself so badly she had to be whisked off to have a shower assisted by Lisa. I'm sure the laughter was therapeutic.

Friends of mine, Natalie and Karen, spent an hour visiting us in the evening. It was great to see them; however, it is amazing how exhausting having visitors can be.

Day three has been another very successful and positive day. My kidney function continues to improve with an eGFR of 54 and a creatinine level of of 105.

Dear Diary,

Day 4 post-transplant...feeling stronger and wireless
3 November 2012

The doctors were very pleased with my continued progress, with my creatinine level having dropped further to 94. I had to keep the catheter in for another full day to take pressure off the bladder sutures. The central intravenous line was removed today, which felt great! It felt as though the nurse picked out four needles that were sitting above my collarbone and then I had to take a deep inhale as he took out some sort of tube. It makes me feel a little queasy thinking about it, but I didn't find it painful.

Mum was always in the bed to the right of me. We both found it frustrating when nurses left the curtain pulled across once they had finished doing our observations. We started to get up and open it up again ourselves, a sign we were getting stronger by the day.

The peripheral intravenous line on the back of my hand was removed today, for which I was grateful as it was becoming uncomfortable.

Dad came up in the afternoon and Tim a little later, in time to watch a bit of Saturday night TV. We had paid to use the TVs that can arch over the beds. It helped to pass the time and kept us resting without getting too bored. I managed to sit in the chair for quite a while and then snuggled as much as possible (with a catheter still inserted between my legs and a sore abdomen) next to Tim on top of my bed. There is a lovely night nurse who would let Tim stay past visiting hours, which usually ended at 8pm! When I started getting uncomfortable, Tim left me to rest, in hope of a good night's sleep.

Dear Diary,

Day 5 post-transplant...DISCHARGE
4 November 2012

I had such trouble getting to sleep last night due to restless legs. I didn't get to sleep until about midnight. I was awake again at 4am, having my blood pressure taken and being asked to drink more water as I was urinating large amounts into the catheter. Luckily, I managed to get back off to sleep again until 6am but woke feeling tired. My blood pressure is still a little on the high side, so they put me back on a low dose of a medication I was taking before the transplant.

I felt disappointed about this as I was keen to not need too many medications post-surgery, but they said I may not be on it forever. I was looking forward to getting the catheter removed today but nervous in case it was uncomfortable. As promised, after the doctors came around, the catheter was taken out. It was slightly undignified, but not a painful experience. I was then asked to pass urine into a jug to monitor the quantity. It soon became clear I would be going to the toilet a lot as I seemed to be passing huge amounts very regularly – approximately 400ml of urine every hour. The quantity was being assessed; therefore, each time, urine needed to be collected in a named jug and left on the side to be recorded. Often, I would worry the jug would not be large enough to contain it all. My hands needed a thorough wash afterwards – I was working on my aim.

The doctors said I could go home today, which I was ecstatic about. The usual hospital stay is seven to ten days for the recipient of a kidney, but my body was healing well, and I couldn't wait to go home to my own bed.

Mummy had a difficult early morning trying to open her bowels and spent an hour on the toilet in a lot of discomfort. However, by 11am she was washed, dressed and ready to go home. She helped me get showered which, after not being able to for five days, felt incredible, even if it was in the hospital ward's basic communal shower cubicle. We sat together for our last lunch at the hospital, watching TV. I started feeling anxious about not getting my drugs in time before the pharmacy closed, which would mean another night on the ward. My mind was so focused on leaving today. I would have been deflated if I couldn't head home.

Dad came up about noon to collect Mum and then left about 1pm after waiting for a while with me. My medications came around 2.30pm and Tim had arrived by then. I was discharged and given instructions about my medications and changing the dressings on my own at home, as well as information about what to look out for regarding blood clots. I also received all necessary contact information for the hospital pharmacy.

Our walk to the transport department in the hospital was slow but smooth and the wait was around twenty minutes for the taxi. I felt nervous about needing the toilet during the journey. I was urinating nearly every thirty minutes. I went to the toilet just before we set off on our bumpy ride. And holy moly was it bumpy! The driver seemed to be heading down every back road with speed ramps. I gripped Tim's hand with one of mine while my other hand clutched against my lower abdomen all the way home – not ideal after major abdominal surgery. The urge to go to the toilet was increasing by the minute. We both asked the driver to slow down. No doubt he was rushing to get back for another job, but these taxis are specifically used for hospital patient transfers. Forty minutes after setting off, we arrived home. Exhausted, exasperated and desperate for the toilet, I clutched my abdomen and climbed the three flights of stairs as fast as I could.

The flat was freezing and all I wanted to do was cry. I'm not sure why I was so emotional suddenly. Maybe I was just relieved to be home or just overwhelmed by the realisation of what we had been through. I felt that my health was still very fragile, and I felt vulnerable now that I wasn't in hospital. After relieving my bladder, some comforting hugs from Tim and a good sleep, I felt more refreshed and ready for dinner.

Tim's mum had popped round just after we got home to bring us a delicious cottage pie with vegetables. It was the best thing I had eaten all week and I polished off some seconds too. She had left a beautiful bunch of flowers and a bottle of Evian water on the lounge table, which was so thoughtful – exactly what I needed. I had a relaxed evening and felt more confident with being discharged and at home as the evening went on.

22

Discharge medication and logbook

Medications at hospital discharge:

Tacrolimus (Advagraf) 6mg every morning

Mycophenolate mofetil 500mg four times a day

Prednisolone 5mg every morning (for one week)

Ranitidine 150mg twice a day

Aspirin 75mg every morning

Co-trimoxazole 480mg every morning

Nystatin 1ml four times a day (one month)

Paracetamol 1g four times a day

Ondansetron 4mg every morning

Amlodipine 5mg every morning

Transplant patient record book or 'blue book'

This book, aptly referred to as the 'blue book' because of its colour, is given to kidney transplant recipients on their day of discharge. It's a logbook for daily fluid intake, blood pressure, temperature, weight, and twenty-four-hour urinary output. Once the catheter is removed, you are asked to collect and measure your urine over a period of twenty-four hours, which gives your specialist a better overall view of your kidney function than one small sample. The specimen jug is easier to aim urine into. This then needs to be poured into the large container also given to you upon discharge.

The book was a reassuring reference for all contact details including transplant nurses, out-of-hours nurses on the ward and hospital transport. It also had pages that could be completed after a clinic appointment, with more information regarding creatinine and haemoglobin levels at each visit, and a section for comments made by the nurse of things to remember. Also, if there was a change in medication, that could be noted too. The blue book and medication list were requested to be taken to every clinic appointment for two months following transplant surgery.

Prescription prepayment certificates (PPCs)

This was something I stumbled upon a month or so following transplant that I wish I had known about beforehand. Transplant medication is not free on the NHS, even though you will be taking it for the rest of your life. There is a list of exemptions for free prescriptions such as if you are sixty or over, under sixteen, pregnant or had a baby in the last twelve months, on income support or an NHS inpatient, to list a few. You can check your eligibility status on the NHS website.

Unfortunately, I didn't meet any of the eligibility criteria. I realised that the prescription prepayment certificate (PPC) would save me a LOT of money! Currently it is £30.25 for three months, or £108.10 for twelve months. The current prescription charge in the UK is £9.35 per item. A little pre-planning can save you money when you run out of the medication you're given when discharged from the hospital.

Part Four

Home Sweet Home

23
Recovery at Home

Dear Diary,

Day 6 post-transplant...
a night from hell and first clinic visit
5 November 2012

Comparing all the nights since the surgery, last night has been the worst. I was in so much pain and constantly having to get up to urinate, nearly every hour. My output total over the last twenty-four hours has been six litres! I ended up sleeping on the sofa as it seemed the only way I could get vaguely comfortable, and I didn't want to disturb Tim. I had an appointment at the clinic in the morning, so I was up by 6.30am and the patient transport arrived at 7.30am. Tim came with me. Both of us were shattered. I knew the first thing I was going to ask the consultant about was my pain management. I had only been given paracetamol! Surely that was not enough?

We got to the clinic and a nurse who had spoken to us about the research project greeted me and explained the procedure of what I needed to do now that I'm attending as a transplant patient. I had some blood taken, along with my weight, and I gave a urine sample. We waited about an hour for my bloods to come through from the lab. At this point I could barely talk and was swaying and leaning forward on the waiting room chair. I felt overwhelmed once my name was called, I couldn't wait to get something for the pain. It was a stressful morning for Tim. He was very quiet and irritable, and I could sense he was tired.

I was seen by the specialist nurse, who has been excellent and who gave me a prescription for a strong pain-relieving drug called tramadol straight away. Tim rushed down to the hospital pharmacy to get this for me. WOW! I'm not sure I have ever experienced pain like that, even in the days after my surgery. I took my first dose of tramadol, and it was a massive relief when it kicked in. The nurse redressed my wound and reassured me that it was very neat. She told me that when the swelling goes down, she will outline where the kidney is situated in my abdomen. The stitches ran from the right side of my lower abdomen (below the level of my navel) down to just above my pubic bone, right through my pubic hair.

I saw Jay and another researcher from the ReMIND research trial, along with the specialist nurse. They all seemed to be happy with the excessive urinating and said it was a very positive sign of a good working kidney.

Tim and I took a steady walk to a London Bridge café and had lunch with a hot chocolate as it was a very cold morning. I thought that maybe I would be allowed a sweet, milky drink now, although I still felt a little naughty for having it.

We got the train home, and I managed to relax in a much more comfortable state. I felt slightly drowsy (a side effect of the medication) but was able to get comfortable. I spent the afternoon on the sofa, very cosy and relaxed. My urinary output has normalised, with a few less trips to the toilet too.

Dear Diary,

Day 8 post-transplant - second clinic visit
7 November 2012

We decided to get the train to the clinic this morning, which was maybe a little ambitious. Our flat was about three hundred metres from New Beckenham train station, and the fast train to London Bridge used to take sixteen minutes. However, I was so slow walking along London Bridge platform that a station assistant asked if we would like a wheelchair to help us get to the hospital. We accepted the help gladly, even though I felt embarrassed and couldn't stop giggling nervously while in the chair.

My abdomen felt very tight and tender this morning. Once inside the hospital and in the renal clinic on Floor 4, Tower Wing, Jay from ReMIND took my bloods for the kidney clinic and his ten bottles for research. I saw a different specialist nurse who checked my blood pressure and found it was slightly low at 100/70. This explained why I felt a little light-headed yesterday when getting up from the sofa!

Everything still seemed to be going very well and the nurse suggested I come off the blood pressure medications. My creatinine level was 103, which she reassured me was good and that it was very rare to have a level under 100 in someone with a transplanted kidney.

The afternoon was very relaxed. Just before bed, I made a trip to the toilet and was really disturbed that my urine had turned a rose colour again. I felt very worried but tried to stay logical. My period was due, and I thought maybe that could be the reason for the colour of my urine. I got up just twice in the night to urinate.

Dear Diary,

Day 10 post-transplant - third clinic visit
9 November 2012

I decided to call the renal clinic yesterday afternoon to get some advice about the rose-coloured urine I continued to have. I got through to a very knowledgeable and experienced renal nurse who was so reassuring. She explained that this was due to bladder irritation by the stent that was inserted to keep my ureter open. It is very common, and it may happen again while I have the stent in. Hopefully it will be removed in about five weeks.

I'm able to lie down more comfortably on my side now. I still get this feeling of fluid around my right lower abdomen, where the transplanted kidney now sits, and it shifts as I move from my side to lying on my back or into a sitting position.

Our journey up to Guy's Hospital was the most comfortable and quickest so far. My blood pressure has improved, and the nurse explained the fluid feeling was due to some fluid surrounding the kidney, which is common. A scan is going to be done at some point next week to check it. The nurse also seemed positive about me doing some gentle abdominal strengthening and ice packs.

Tim devised a rehab programme for me (being a physiotherapist, this was right up his street) and we went through it when we got back home. I did some hot and cold packs and gentle massage into my abdomen and groin. I'm keen to see if it helps.

Dear Diary,

Day 11 post-transplant – a day with family and Mum
10 November 2012

I have much less sensation of that fluid movement in my lower abdomen already. Sitting up in bed before going to the toilet is less painful, so I'm going to keep on with my rehab along with the hot and cold packing.

I was looking forward to seeing my two aunts, Lisa and Jan, who were going over to Mum and Dad's for the afternoon. Tim dropped me off on his way to work. When I arrived, Mum and Dad were sitting in bed. Mum felt a little lethargic, which is how she has been pretty much all week. She has embraced loafing about and tends to lie in bed all morning and lie on the sofa the rest of the day. I'm not sure it's good, mentally, to do that and it can make you feel more lethargic. Dad is doing absolutely everything for her, which again, I'm not sure is so helpful. For me, I have gained something my body really needed and I feel like I am starting to thrive. For Mum, her body has lost an organ and I think that is a challenge for her body to adapt to. It's about finding a balance between activity and rest. Not doing enough for yourself fails to challenge and strengthen you, but the mind often overrules any motivation to be active.

One of my closest friends, Hannah, came over to my parents with her newborn baby just after noon as she lives nearby. Mum and I had a little cuddle with the baby. My aunts arrived shortly after.

Lisa washed and blow-dried my hair, which was such a treat. It was so uplifting to spend time with my family and friend, and I think it perked Mum up too. She just seemed a little low in mood and I wasn't sure what to say. I mean, I couldn't tell her to cheer up. After all, she was put in this situation of pain and discomfort because of me and only me.

Dear Diary,

Day 17 post-transplant - fourth clinic visit
16 November 2012

Many of my days are very similar now, relaxed and steady. This week has been good though, with progress and good feedback at my appointments, which are still three times a week. I have managed to sleep all through the night over the last two nights. I have been advised by one of the renal specialist nurses that as long as I'm taking in 2–2.5 litres a day, I don't need to be drinking during the night. It has worked beautifully, and I didn't get up to go to the toilet until 7am.

I went to spend the afternoon at Mum and Dad's, which was nice. Mum was a little tired, but it was nice to give her a little cuddle. Tim's mum came to the clinic with me one day this week, which I think she found interesting, and it was nice to have the company. My best day so far this week was when my friends from the Tonbridge clinic, Nicola and Gemma, came to visit. They brought me some lovely flowers, sweeties and smellies. They were really shocked at how well I was looking, and how trim I looked and felt when they gave me a cuddle. It was lovely to get some positive feedback. Lots of my patients have been asking after me, with at least one call from one of them every day asking the clinic receptionists for an update. I am touched at how caring and concerned my patients have been.

My appointment went well today. In fact, I am getting the uncomfortable bladder stent out next week. My creatinine level is 107, and my blood pressure is 100/70, which I was very pleased about, and my dressing can now be removed. I had a clearer explanation about the location of the kidney, which was described as superficial to the intestines in the lower abdomen and to the right of the bladder. I also asked the nurse about the position of the kidney if I were to become pregnant (God willing at some point in the future). Apparently, as the uterus expands, the kidney would continue to move to the right to accommodate the growth of the uterus.

In general, my posture is really improving, and I can walk as fast as any other commuter in town now. My face has become thinner and my skin is a lot less spotty. The girls made me laugh during their visit, as they admitted to thinking I looked a little yellow before the transplant!

Dear Diary,

Day 20 post-transplant - clinic visit, stent removal day
19 November 2012

I woke up today feeling nervous about the procedure this afternoon. I had a check-up at the renal clinic first, so Tim and I made our way there. The train was blissfully quiet. As soon as I got to the hospital, I felt light-headed and when my blood pressure was done, it was recording as 91/63. I wasn't sure why it was so low, but it explained why my head felt very strange. My appointment went well apart from that, and the renal nurse suggested I try and drink a little more fluid as I struggle to take in much more than what I pass.

Tim and I went for a pub lunch in London Bridge as my stent removal wasn't until the afternoon. I decided to have a big warming lunch and went completely out of character with my choice of a cheeseburger and French fries. It tasted great!! I thought maybe it

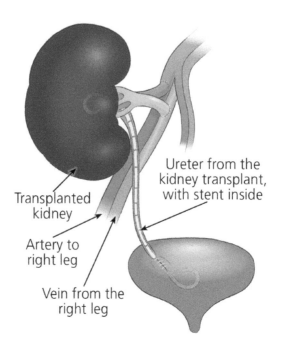

Transplanted
kidney

Ureter from the
kidney transplant,
with stent inside

Artery to
right leg

Vein from the
right leg

*The image above shows the stent inside the ureter from a transplanted
kidney to the bladder.*

*would help to increase my low blood pressure too. I felt better after
eating, but maybe that was due to the trio of desserts that we shared!
It is so good to not have to be so strict with what I eat. I'm loving the
ability, to once again, eat dairy guilt-free.*

*I was feeling really nervous about this stent removal by the time
we got back to the hospital. There was a young guy wearing a white
coat sitting outside the room I was due to go in. Once the doctor
arrived, I realised the young guy was a medical student. I thought...Oh.
My. God! Not only is the doctor doing the procedure male, a blinking
male student wants to peer at my vagina while the procedure is being
done. My hands became very sweaty. A female nurse came out and
asked if I would be comfortable with the student being in there. All I
could visualise were two men peering at my private bits with my legs*

open. So no, I wouldn't be comfortable! The student came outside and sat back where he was sitting. I felt a little guilty, but it was traumatic enough having the thing done. They called me in.

After a painful antibiotic injection in my right thigh, for which I was neither prepared nor briefed about beforehand, I had to assume the usual 'smear position' (for any chaps reading this, this is lying on your back, with your feet together and knees opened wide). It's so undignified and embarrassing. It's bad enough with a female nurse but I just had to block out the male doctor wiping my vagina with saline and antiseptic, then injecting some sort of anaesthetic up there. A long, black instrument called a cystoscope was handed to him by the nurse. He proceeded to insert this instrument up my urethra and into my bladder, instantly causing my pelvic floor muscles to go rigid and causing severe discomfort. I looked up at the ceiling and tried my hardest to relax. He then threaded some form of wire or tube along the scope. I was afraid to look. I could imagine he was trying to hook onto the stent. I suddenly felt an uncomfortable tugging and my urethra being stretched while the scope, along with the stent, was on its way back out. Thank God for that!! I couldn't get my clothes on quickly enough. Oddly, all I could feel was my painful right thigh, which felt as though someone had just punched it really hard.

I had a little whimper outside the room with Tim. I suddenly didn't feel so bad about my choice of not allowing the student to observe. The procedure was every bit as traumatic as I had imagined it would be. I was just glad it was over. Tim got me home with a hot chocolate in my hands. I got a little teary while telling Mum about it on the phone. I'm not sure why I felt quite so emotional. It may have been because it was around such a sensitive and private area of my body. On reflection, I realised that it was over and done with in less than a couple of minutes, which I am grateful for.

Dear Diary,

Day 24 - 3 weeks post-transplant
23 November 2012

I started my period today, so yesterday's emotional episode is explained. I was still a little worried about the colour change of my urine. However, it felt great to think my body was starting to get back to normal and my menstrual cycle was getting back into sync.

My appointment went well; I feel well, and my proteinuria has improved. My haemoglobin remains low, but the consultant is happy with my iron stores. I've been very satisfied with the care at Guy's Hospital. It's an easy commute and I have three clinic visits each week.

Medications 3 weeks post-transplant:

Tacrolimus (Advagraf) 6mg every morning

Mycophenolate mofetil 1g twice a day

Co-trimoxazole 480mg every morning

Aspirin 75mg every morning

Omeprazole 20mg twice a day

Tramadol as needed

Dear Diary,

8 weeks post-transplant
28 December 2012

Wow! I can't believe it's nearly 8 weeks since my kidney transplant. Looking back, there have been lots of exciting events, including my thirtieth birthday and Christmas, and my new kidney continues to function well. My creatinine level seems to fluctuate between 103umol/L and 119umol/L. I much prefer it when it's closer to 100 as I feel it's as good as it can possibly be. I am on one appointment per week now at Guy's Hospital. The doctors and nurses are all pleased that I am doing so well, and Jay mentioned that I have one of the best functioning kidneys of those who had recent transplants at the hospital. Go, kidney!

I had such an amazing thirtieth birthday with a surprise party organised by my wonderful Tim. I didn't have a clue. Even though I was in five-inch heels and standing all night, I felt so energised and alive! I was home and in bed by 12.30am but I don't think I managed to get to sleep until about 2am with the endorphin rush and reflecting on what a wonderful night it had been. I had lots of family and friends there celebrating with me and my first glass of champagne since the transplant.

I have struggled a little this month with restless legs and light, disturbed sleep. I have concluded that this occurs when I haven't done enough physical activity during the day. I really do feel well now – my energy level is so much higher and I have no abdominal pain. I have taken the odd tramadol just to help with getting to sleep but knowing how addictive tramadol is, I have decided to only take it as necessary for pain. I just need to do more exercise now and use up all this newfound energy I have before bedtime.

I decided to spend Christmas lunch with Tim, his mum and sister. I think it might have helped distract from the fact that this year was the first Christmas without Tim's dad, Richard. It was always going to be awful, with or without me, but I just wanted to be there to help in some way. I did tire myself out by driving to Swindon in the late afternoon. It made me acutely aware that my body still needs a little more time to recover. I have been a little torn by all the Christmas celebrating and still having to limit my intake of alcohol. I know that my first priority is to protect this gift of life I have been blessed to receive. I have kept really hydrated and increased my water intake while having an alcoholic drink. If I can keep that up as a habit, I think it's acceptable for me to have an occasional glass of spirits. I would like to recommend to anyone with CKD, before and after transplant, that it is of paramount importance to follow your doctor's instructions regarding alcohol consumption.

Tonbridge clinic had a lovely Christmas meal, and I was so happy to be able to attend. All my colleagues complimented me on how well I was looking. They asked me when I might be coming back to work. My heart would like to go back early in January, but my mind overrules my heart. I'm thinking I should give it until the end of January, which would be three months post-transplant. I am planning to use the early part of January to get stronger with some core stability exercise and cardio. I need to do more in the New Year as the festivities will be over and I'll end up pondering on my thoughts with too much time on my hands.

Mummy is back to her old self now and planning to go back to work on light duties without too much lifting in early January 2013.

Medications 8 weeks post-transplant:

Tacrolimus (Advagraf) 6mg once a day

Mycophenolate mofetil 1g twice a day

Co-trimoxazole 480mg once a day

Aspirin 75mg once a day

24

Three months post-transplant

I WAS STILL DOING WELL THREE MONTHS after surgery and went back to work very part-time. I also started baking at home, just to fill a void and have something to do to pass the time. It was at this point I decided enough was enough. I needed to get back to work! I desperately needed to regain my sense of purpose by doing what I loved. I wanted to earn some money again too! I was renting a flat with Tim and, luckily, he was happy to cover my expenses while I was unable to work.

My latest lab results were very good. My eGFR was 56; my blood pressure was 118/76 and I had a heart rate of 81. My weight dropped following the transplant to 58.8kg, from around 62–63kg pre-transplant, so I had lost about 4–5kg in weight, most probably fluid retention. I had weekly appointments to make sure my tacrolimus level was within the target range of 3–7ug/L. The bloods taken to give an accurate reading needed to be around twelve hours after the last dose taken. I had to start mentally noting to not take it on the morning of my appointment as it was starting to become habitual in my morning routine by this point.

Diet and fluid intake

It really was so wonderful to not feel restricted by any special diets. I have always been a healthy eater, and I was so happy to get back to having the foods I felt were healthy.

I really had to keep up with the water intake. I bought packs of six two-litre mineral water bottles, which I would get through in a week, along with other drinks during the day. I didn't leave the house without some sort of water bottle in my bag. The colour of my urine was my guide to whether I was drinking enough. Almost translucent was what I was working towards.

25

Six months post-transplant

AFTER FOUR MONTHS, MY TRANSPLANT follow-up appointments were bi-weekly. My bloods and blood pressure were great, so I began doing some cycling again. I was feeling well – so much stronger and I had lots more energy. I had no swelling after the longer bike rides and felt that setting the challenge of cycling to Paris may be achievable now that I had a healthy functioning kidney.

I felt passionate about raising money for Guy's and St Thomas' Charity as a thank you for all that the staff had done for me. The care and expertise Mum and I experienced was incredible. So Tim and I set a date to cycle from London to Paris – the early May bank holiday weekend of 2013. I started telling family and friends and work patients all about our plan and they were extremely supportive and generous with their sponsorship donations. My parents were a little apprehensive, as it was only six months after having major surgery. I tried to reassure them I was feeling up to it. In all honesty, I really wasn't sure that I could do it. This was going to be a three-day cycle of over two hundred miles (gulp!). What I *was* sure of was that I had to try. I had sponsorship donations coming in thick and fast leading up to our departure date, and I just didn't want to let anybody down!

I was more than just a little nervous about how my kidney would cope during a cycle ride of this length. I had cycled forty miles two days running just two weeks prior and felt well, with no change in my kidney function. That really boosted my confidence!!

26
London-to-Paris bike ride for GSTT Charity

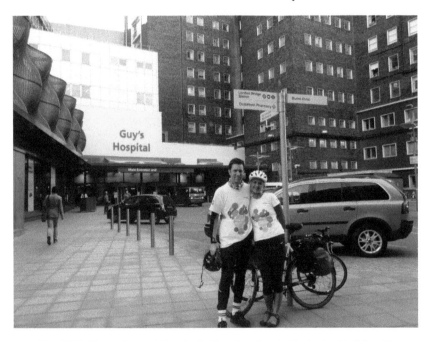

May 2012, Tim and me at the start of our London-to-Paris charity bike ride.
Seven months post-surgery.

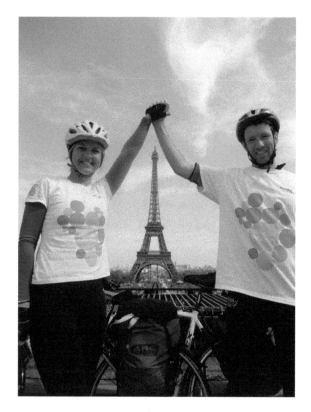

Tim and me at the finish line.
The Eiffel Tower in Paris. We cycled 222 miles over three days.

Seven months post-transplant

We set off on 2 May 2013 outside Guy's Hospital. Our starting time: 7.30am. The weather was beautifully sunny, and we seemed to get out of London in no time. Our route took us past St George's Hospital in Tooting – where my kidney disease was first diagnosed – down through Godstone and Guildford, and then the toughest part, through the South Downs.

A few times during my training I had developed knee pain and worried that this might hinder me on the ride. My knee did start to play up and there were a few steep hills I had to walk the bike up. We arrived in Portsmouth by about 6pm and managed to get on the overnight ferry to Le Havre around 11pm. Mum and Dad met us in Portsmouth to offer support. I didn't mention anything regarding my knee. I put on my brave (but tired) face. That evening, I took a strong painkiller, tramadol, which was left over from the transplant surgery and did lots of ice packs on my knee. I was worried about how I would get through day two.

We were graced with fine, sunny weather in France and set off around 8.30am. It was a slow morning trying to figure out our best route out of the port towards Paris. We rode through some beautiful villages with magnificent sights and this seemed to help distract from the enormity of the hills we were climbing! The painkiller that I took helped, and when cycling on the flat roads, I could barely feel a thing.

Tired and settling in Évreux for the night after another nine hours of cycling, we managed to have a nice hot bath and some supper to recharge before our final day of cycling (fingers crossed)!

Day three came, and we set off early, making great progress as the roads were flatter on this last leg. We finally arrived in Paris around 5pm, the Eiffel Tower our finish line. I felt a little sad that our journey had come to an end, as I can truly say I loved every minute of it.

We really enjoyed the challenge and were so fortunate to be blessed with wonderful weather, and the views in both countries were outstanding. I felt so very lucky to have been able to do this bike ride. It would not have been possible without the care and skills of the staff at Guy's Hospital. We managed to raise just over £1,500 for Guy's and St Thomas' Charity.

At seven to eight months I was having monthly post-transplant clinic appointments. I was taken off aspirin, which pleased me greatly as I had been bruising like a peach! Hopefully, that would improve! Mycophenolate mofetil (MMF) was decreased due to a change in my white blood cell count.

Medications 8 months post-transplant:

Tacrolimus (Advagraf) 6mg once a day

Mycophenolate mofetil 250mg twice a day

Co-trimoxazole 480mg once a day

27

Post-transplant skin surveillance clinic

12 months post-transplant

The post-transplant skin surveillance clinic in the dermatology department is fantastic at Guy's Hospital. I had a mole on my back that I was unsure about and wanted checked, and I got a referral straight away. Anti-rejection medications increase the risk of cancerous skin lesions, including melanoma. This was all explained in the clinic, along with the importance of using a high SPF sunscreen. I was a sun worshipper in my teens and early twenties and had also used sun beds (tut tut!), so this was a real wake-up call to look after my skin. I headed down to the shops and stocked up on SPF 50!

Fortunately, the mole I had on my back was nothing abnormal, and since then I have had a yearly full body dermatological inspection. I find this reassuring and such a great preventative approach. I also had my facial acne evaluated. I've had occasional acne on and off since my teens. The doctor assured me that this was nothing serious and suggested a topical gel to treat it.

Medications 12 months post-transplant:

Tacrolimus (Advagraf) 6mg once a day

Mycophenolate mofetil 250mg twice a day

28

Renal pre-pregnancy planning clinic

AS I PASSED THE ONE-YEAR ANNIVERSARY of my transplant, my goal was to begin focusing on starting a family. I was referred to the pre-pregnancy counselling clinic. Tim and I discussed the prospect of having a baby and he seemed happy. In fact, I think it must have got him thinking a lot about starting a family. He proposed to me in February, sixteen months following the transplant.

The pre-pregnancy counselling clinic felt like a VIP service and was such a privilege. We shared a room with my renal consultant, who I knew well by now, along with an obstetric physician and a consultant obstetrician. Three highly skilled medical professionals all interested in helping to support me. Wow! Yet again I felt very lucky. After looking at my history and renal transplant, my blood tests and blood pressure, they concluded that I could indeed begin trying to conceive. This really did feel like my next personal challenge.

I was warned that there was a risk that my creatinine level would rise during pregnancy and remain at an elevated baseline following delivery, but the risk of significant damage to my transplanted kidney, either during or after pregnancy, was very low.

I felt the risk-to-reward ratio was in favour of having a baby. The MMF medication would need to be switched to azathioprine two to three months prior to starting to try to conceive. Mycophenolate mofetil is associated with a 20–25 per cent risk of foetal abnormalities, and is unsafe to take during the first trimester.

It was also explained that I was at increased risk for pre-eclampsia due to my history of renal disease. The associated risks of premature delivery and necessity for C-section were also factors. I would need to start a 75mg dose of aspirin once a day to reduce the risk, along with folic acid. When discussing the C-section, a transplant surgeon advised a midline skin incision and transverse uterine incision to help reduce the risk of damage to the transplanted kidney. All the literature I read quoted a 1–2 per cent risk of damage to the graft during a caesarean section.

This was all fantastic preparation! We were enjoying the planning and celebrations for our upcoming wedding, and so happy to be able to plan for our future!

29

Canada and the cystitis attack

TRAVEL WAS ON THE AGENDA THE YEAR following transplant, to visit my cousin working at the Banff Springs Hotel in Canada. After the busy build-up and over-consumption of Christmas, a couple of weeks in the snowy Rocky Mountains sounded perfect! I felt fit and well, and my bloods were stable and coming back with great results. The consultants were happy with me, and I had all this energy and zest for life, my gift of life post-transplant! After numerous hours learning how to ski on the dry slopes of Orpington, we flew into Calgary on 28 December 2013.

We were queuing at passport control and I got the strangest feeling that I urgently needed to urinate. Afterwards, I felt a horrid burning sensation, then the sense of urgency again. This did not feel comfortable in the slightest. We were travelling to Banff from Calgary in a hire car, and there were so many times on our journey I had to stop. I started drinking lots and lots of water. I was aware that I hadn't drank enough fluids on our flight. While I had never had cystitis, I had heard and read about it while studying for my osteopathy degree. *This must be it!* I thought.

I wasn't sure how I was going to get treated. I needed to call a doctor in Canada quickly, but where would I start? I had such a wave of panic come over me like never before. I felt so worried for my new kidney transplant. I couldn't chance this infection making its way up to my new precious kidney, which was so much closer to my bladder. I had stupidly forgotten to get travel insurance before leaving London. What an idiot! This was going to cost me big time!

We managed to get a call-out doctor to come to the hotel room. I felt like I couldn't leave the room for fear of needing the loo so frequently. He took a urine sample from me and gave me a four-day prescription for co-amoxiclav and a probiotic to protect my intestinal flora while on the antibiotic – very forward-thinking on his part.

It was a day or so after taking them that I started to feel more comfortable. The doctor called me the following day explaining there was bacteria in the urine sample, so I am glad I had started the antibiotics quickly. A juicy £500-plus bill really did drum it into me never to go away without travel insurance. I was fully covered by 29 December!

Recurrent cystitis

By the time I returned from Canada and was back in for my renal follow-up, the symptoms of cystitis were back. I was given a different antibiotic to try called ciprofloxacin. It was frustrating to have it come back so soon. I had been taking co-trimoxazole for a whole year following transplant surgery, which is a medication used to treat bacterial infections such as those in the urinary tract. I wasn't taking this anymore and wondered if I was I more susceptible to picking up UTIs now.

I had frequent episodes of cystitis throughout 2014, often taking antibiotics. I wasn't particularly happy about this, as I know that overuse of antibiotics can cause bacteria to become resistant to treatment. I became very analytical about what was causing these horrible attacks. We were using condoms during intercourse and I became obsessed about personal hygiene. I frequently had loose bowel movements, which a renal consultant mentioned can contribute to the transfer of bacteria to the bladder. The MMF medication can cause side effects of diarrhoea, but obviously I needed to take this for anti-rejection purposes.

I tried everything I had read about avoiding cystitis and UTIs. I would spend more time sitting on the toilet, as it was suggested that incomplete emptying of the bladder and urinary retention can cause irritation. I was also told to empty my bladder after intercourse.

I ended up getting four episodes of cystitis throughout this year, even one just before our wedding in September. This was unfortunate timing to say the least. That particular episode I linked to drinking coffee a day or two beforehand. Whether that had been an irritant to the bladder, I wasn't sure. These bouts of cystitis were a bit of a mystery to me, as at least two of them showed no bacterial growth. The subsequent episodes caused some discomfort when urinating as well as increased urinary frequency. Interestingly, over that same period, I suffered with intermittent headaches accompanied by nausea and vomiting. Maybe wedding preparation stress had a significant part to play in all these symptoms.

Bladder scans had come back normal and it was suggested I self-start antibiotics (amoxicillin) if cystitis symptoms recurred. I felt disappointed with the amount of antibiotics I had needed over this year, but at the same time I felt more anxious about a urinary tract infection, which could possibly lead to infection in my donor kidney. I was taking food supplements to help with the urinary symptoms. These included D-Mannose, cranberry extract and probiotics.

Part Five

Motherhood and More

30

Pregnancy with a kidney transplant

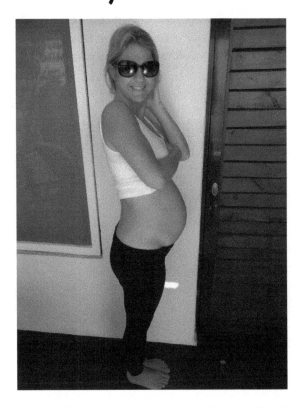

May 2015. Twenty-five weeks pregnant in Crete. Showing off my bump and smaller 'kidney bump', which moved sideways as my tummy expanded.

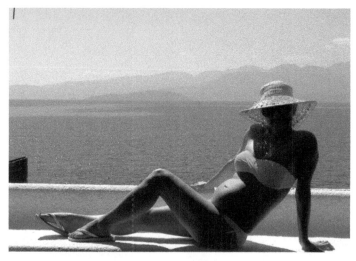

Twenty-five weeks pregnant in Elounda, Crete. Factor 50 sunscreen on and feeling warm, excited and blessed.

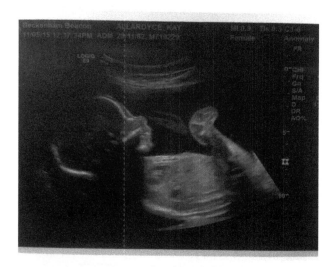

May 2015. Twenty-two-week scan performed at the Beckenham Beacon hospital. No abnormalities were noted – what a huge relief.

Big changes...

By the end of September, we were married and we set off on our honeymoon to India in late December. I had some increased urinary frequency while travelling and made frequent toilet visits while on a ten-hour train ride from Hospet to Kochi. It was tricky, aiming into a hole in the floor of one of the carriages while squatting on a bumpy train, but it all added to the honeymoon story. By the time we were back, I realised it had been a few weeks since having any cystitis symptoms. I had skipped a period and YES...I was PREGNANT!

Pregnancy with a transplant

I had switched my medications from MMF to azathioprine after we got married in September. We waited three months before heading to India for our honeymoon. We couldn't have planned it any better! I got pregnant on our honeymoon!

The sun was warming 'Mini' and me while we enjoyed the view of Poro Bay, Elounda, on the island of Crete. I was excited and grateful for this magical feeling that a little person was growing day by day inside me. With every flutter and movement, I felt the wonder and anticipation of who this little person would be! And all the while, I felt so calm and relaxed. We called the bump Mini (cheesy, I know!). The SPF 50 covered every inch of me while I lay on a lounger under the parasol on the terrace of our room. I relished in the beauty and love of being pregnant, having a baby bump I didn't have to hide under clothes, and breasts I never had before that looked great in a bodycon dress! I felt well – no sickness. My kidney was working well and Mini was growing perfectly. Life was great.

Breaking the news to Mum and Dad

It was February 2015, and Mum and I were standing in a little narrow office within the industrial kitchen of Meals on Wheels, Wallington branch, where she worked. I would often pop in if I had a gap between patients, who I saw in the clinic down the road. She seemed very excited about the news my brother and his fiancée were due to get married in October and started talking about getting some flights booked for all four of us to attend. My due date was the end of September! I was only a couple of months pregnant, but I had to tell her there was no way I could go to the wedding as I would have just given birth!

We hugged and she laughed with excitement, but I felt sorry for my parents that these two life events were happening so close together. The excitement quickly switched to concern that the kidney was functioning well enough and would be okay while I was pregnant. I reassured her and Dad when I saw him later that day. Worry and what-if scenarios always seem to come first before a follow-up reaction of excitement with Dad. I was glad they now knew. Trying to keep it quiet for another month was going to be a challenge.

Scans of the baby and kidney

I had more scans than a typical pregnancy, more so in the last trimester (twenty-seven weeks onwards). I really didn't mind in the slightest and looked forward to them. Each time I saw this wonderful little person growing and moving around, I couldn't help but feel reassured that they were snuggled up next to Mum's donated kidney. Without her sacrifice, it would have been impossible to experience and carry this wonderful gift of my baby. It was like having a check-in on the kidney each time too, as this gift had always been my priority. After my pregnancy, it would be my priority again!

Health and wellbeing while pregnant

Throughout the forty weeks of my pregnancy, I was continually assessing the growth and health of the baby, as well as the equally important health and function of my one working donated kidney.

I knew about healthy living, as this was part of my naturopathic training at university. I was determined to get as close to full term as I could, making healthy lifestyle choices in order to have a healthy pregnancy and a healthy baby. I already worked part-time, so I continued seeing patients and eliminated the heavier manual techniques I had used previously. I took time to relax and meditate, and although I continued to teach Pilates until about thirty weeks into my pregnancy, I began pregnancy yoga and Pilates classes outside of work. I felt strong, happy and healthy, a perfect combination while pregnant. My diet was clean, and I didn't feel like drinking alcohol at all. I found it incredible that growing another human can totally change your mindset on what you choose to consume or not.

I investigated HypnoBirthing after finding a flyer in the maternity clinic at Beckenham Beacon. Janice Champion is a yoga instructor, midwife and HypnoBirthing instructor. What a woman! I had to meet her and learn this skill. Tim was completely up for it too. We both agreed that if I could try and give birth naturally (vaginally), then there was less chance of a C-section incision damaging the kidney which, as mentioned, can happen in a small number of emergency C-sections, due to the location of the kidney in the pelvis.

HypnoBirthing is an approach to safe, easier and more comfortable birthing. It helps manage pain using visualisations, relaxation and breathing techniques. We used visualisations of the uterus moving the baby through the birth canal during a contraction, using the breathing to control the sensations. Directed breathing while the baby is coming out helps to avoid tearing and keeps the flow of labour going. It was empowering, and it gave Tim some things to be working on to keep me relaxed and in the zone. I had affirmations to listen to and recite daily, embedding these into my mind, things like "I put all fear aside as I prepare for the birth of my baby," and "My muscles work in complete harmony to make birthing easier." Visualising the anatomy and the physiological changes really helped keep my mind focused on birthing as an unfolding experience, and it took the fear away. In fact, I felt excited!

I also worked on perineal stretching, using a device called an EPI-NO, which had claimed to reduce the risk of tearing by over forty per cent. I used it after week thirty-seven and coincided using it with doing my affirmation work.

Medication during pregnancy #1

I continued taking tacrolimus and azathioprine, which remained the same dosage throughout my pregnancy. In addition, I was taking folic acid and aspirin. At sixteen weeks into my pregnancy, there were signs that I was becoming anaemic. I was prescribed Mircera (erythropoietin) again and given an intravenous iron infusion to boost my iron stores.

31
Giving birth to George

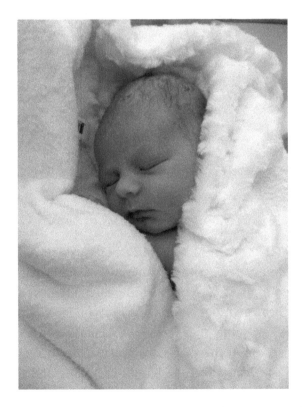

George Richard Patrick Allardyce. Born 18 September 2015. A few hours old, wrapped in a blanket gifted to us by my godmother, Sandra Morgan.

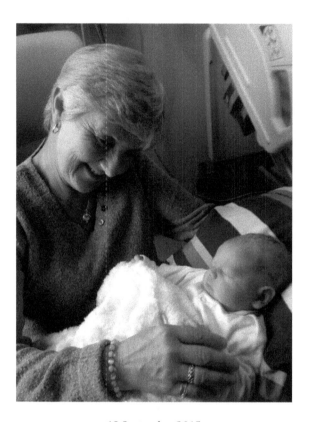

18 September 2015.
Mum meeting George for the first time.

I GAVE BIRTH TO A HEALTHY BABY boy three days prior to my expected delivery date, with no pain relief or medical intervention. We managed to use the HypnoBirthing techniques and my labour was not a long drawn-out affair. I was grateful for not needing pain relief as this can sometimes be known to make you feel woozy or sick. Also if some of the drugs are given close to delivery, there is a chance they can affect the baby's breathing and possibly the first feed. I sustained a second-degree perineal tear, which was left to heal on its own. To say I was happy and relieved was an understatement.

I really pushed for a water birth, but due to the need for continuous foetal monitoring, I couldn't. I used all my HypnoBirthing techniques on the bed, in the maternity ward and sat on the maternity ball whenever I could. Giving birth on all fours seemed to really make sense to me, with gravity working with the baby's descent, so I used this position most of the time. My labour was short at just under three hours.

My blood pressure had just started to creep up in the last week of pregnancy. The consultants were happy that I was beyond the thirty-seven-week threshold and felt the baby was comfortably 'cooked'. I was diagnosed with pre-eclampsia, showing some protein in my urine, an elevated blood pressure and a creatinine level of 139. The midwife tried to initiate labour with a stretch and sweep as part of an internal vaginal examination. This on its own didn't get labour started so I had a hormonal pessary inserted, and within a few hours I was having regular contractions. I gave birth to George Richard Patrick at 2.42am, with him weighing 7lb 4oz.

32
Breastfeeding

I WAS VERY FORTUNATE TO HAVE Kate Bramham as my consultant nephrologist, who also runs a specialist renal-pregnancy service at King's College Hospital and is lead for the UK Renal Disease in Pregnancy study group.

Kate, along with others, wrote a paper on breastfeeding and tacrolimus whereby they assessed the tacrolimus levels in breast milk and neonatal exposure during breastfeeding. The conclusion made was that tacrolimus ingested by infants via breast milk is negligible and women taking this medication should not be discouraged from breastfeeding.

This was music to my ears. I knew that breastfeeding would offer so many amazing benefits to the baby, and to me. I thought I would list them as they amaze me each time.

The benefits of breastfeeding:

- Breast milk protects your baby from infections and diseases.
- Your breast milk is designed for your baby and is available whenever your baby needs it.

- Breastfeeding can build a strong emotional bond between you and your baby.

Breastfeeding and the production of breast milk have benefits for the mother too, and the more you feed, the greater the benefits. Breastfeeding can lower your risk of obesity, cardiovascular disease, osteoporosis and breast and ovarian cancers. It seemed like a no-brainer for me to breastfeed, especially since I'm taking immunosuppressant medications for the rest of my life! Breastfeeding can naturally boost my immune system to fight all these diseases.

Unfortunately, breastfeeding was incredibly painful for the first couple of weeks. I placed refrigerated cabbage leaves on my breasts and rubbed lanolin on my nipples after every feed. But it was so worth it. Each feed offered such special quiet time, and lots of bonding with cuddles. Oh, and we got through the whole *Breaking Bad* box set in a couple of months, and not a penny spent on milk.

About ten days after having my son, I found he just wasn't latching on and I panicked. I had heard about breastfeeding cafés at the NCT course we had attended and so I packed up my baby bag and took my crying baby to the closest one, which was in Penge in southeast London, right next to the train station. It was in a basic public hall, with lots of chairs available, all situated in a circular-style gathering. New mums and 'established' mums, all with their breasts out and feeding babies (or not, as the case was for me). This incredibly calm, friendly woman who ran the club was a lactation specialist – 'angel in disguise' – who came around to me. She positioned my baby's head and me in such a way he latched on straight away. What a feeling of relief! I breastfed George for twelve months. I would highly recommend these cafés. They are critical for new mums who want to breastfeed.

It's completely true that no one can prepare you for having your own child. I often found myself very tired, which I presumed was due to sleep deprivation and I knew I wasn't managing to drink half as much as I had been drinking prior to giving birth.

I did get a bit of a blip in my kidney function with my creatinine rising to 172umol/L a month after giving birth. It was suspected that I was dehydrated and not drinking enough fluids. I also had a bout of mastitis and was given a course of antibiotics. I had read that breastfeeding can help clear the milk duct blockage that may have led to the infection in the first place, so I kept breastfeeding. I did lots of breast pumping too, and lots of crying as it was very painful. I generally felt really poorly as well because I had a fever. Luckily it didn't last more than a week. Four weeks later my creatinine was back on track at 128umol/L, which was my pre-pregnancy baseline. I was very pleased. I was seen monthly at the clinic for five months, then the intervals increased again to once every three to four months.

33
Giving birth to Rosealin

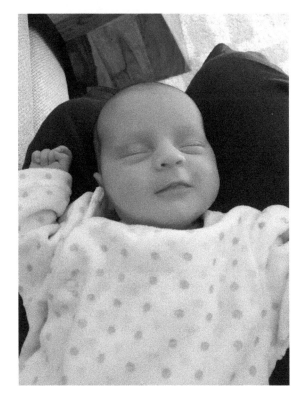

Our beautiful Rosealin Margaret Allardyce.
Born 18 August 2017.

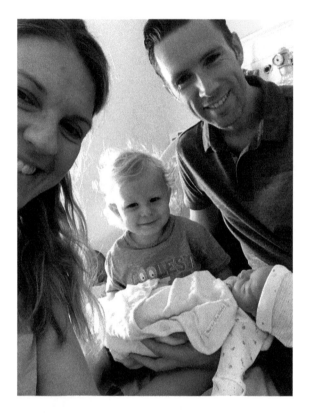

19 August 2017. King's College Hospital maternity ward.
The moment George met his little sister, Rosealin.

ROSEALIN MARGARET WAS BORN a year and eleven months after George. My pregnancy was a little shorter due to pre-eclampsia again, and I delivered at thirty-five weeks. I went for my obstetric check-up appointment straight after a morning of treating patients. I had no idea that three days later, Rosealin would be born! My blood pressure was unbelievably high, and there was protein in my urine again. I had no symptoms and would never have known. I was put on a medication called nifedipine, but it didn't decrease my blood pressure adequately. The medics felt the best solution was to deliver the baby.

I was put in an ambulance from Princess Royal University Hospital and 'blue lighted' to King's College Hospital, which did no favours for my blood pressure whatsoever. Once there, I was examined and given a sweep and stretch. They wanted to break my waters, which I felt strongly against and wanted to try the hormone pessary again like I had used with my first baby. Once again this was enough to start my labour. I quickly got into the HypnoBirthing mindset. Eight hours later, at 7.37am, Rosealin was born, weighing 6lb 2oz.

During the pregnancy I received erythropoietin therapy again for anaemia, and my tacrolimus dose was raised slightly to 7mg. I also took a low dose of aspirin. I continued nifedipine, 10mg twice daily, for a few months until my blood pressure settled. I still had some proteinuria three months following delivery, but my creatinine level returned to 128umol/L, which was my pre-pregnancy level. I was elated to think my kidney hadn't been stressed too much.

Interestingly, by eight months after delivery, my creatinine level had slowly climbed to around 130–40umol/L. I was being seen every three to four months. I continued to breastfeed until Rosealin was thirteen months old and stayed on azathioprine. There was some discussion about returning to mycophenolate once I finished breastfeeding. However, as I had a low white cell count while on mycophenolate and my transplant was classed as being immunologically low risk, it was decided that I was not to switch over for the time being.

34
Life with two

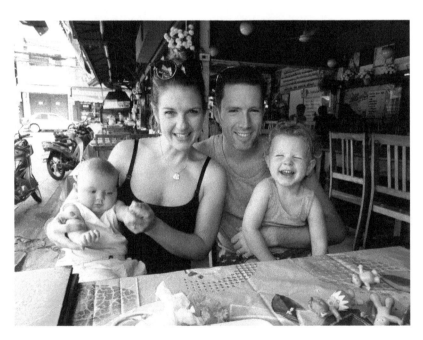

Tim, George (age 2) and Rosealin (4 months) in Ko Samui, Thailand.
January 2018.

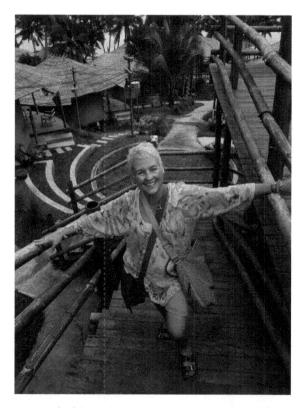

My wonderful Auntie Lisa with us in Ko Samui, Thailand.

I WAS TIRED, AS ANY MOTHER OF two young children would be, but I felt well, and my blood pressure was well-controlled at about 128/88. I felt I had achieved a personal goal that I had been aiming for. I'm so grateful that my body has coped so well with two pregnancies and childbirths. I have a feeling that trying to have a third child would be pushing my luck. This kidney needs to last me as long as possible, and I can't help but feel that the added stress of another pregnancy and childbirth could cause permanent damage. I owe it to my children and my husband to be present in their lives for as long as I possibly can.

Seven years post-transplant, my tacrolimus brand was switched from Advagraf (taken once a day) to Adoport (taken twice a day) due to cost savings for the NHS. It was disappointing as my medication schedule was so simple. Getting up in the morning and taking the two medications together with a pint of water was so easy, then I didn't have to think about it again until the following day. However, this change meant that I needed to remember that second dose in the early evening, roughly twelve hours following the morning dose. I needed to learn a new habit, but to this day I still forget occasionally and find myself getting out of bed to take that second dose before going to sleep.

Travels with two...

We took an incredible family trip to Thailand just four months after Rosealin was born. It was a bit daunting, as the trip had been pre-booked, and I wasn't sure how I would be feeling. That same wonderful aunt who was beside me post-transplant came with us. Her extra pair of hands were a godsend with two small children!

I was feeling well and had a fantastic experience. It was great being away from the UK during the hard month of January. I stayed super hydrated, slathered on the SPF 50 and took plenty of my anti-rejection meds. The area we visited didn't require any vaccinations. 'Live' vaccines are to be avoided if you've had an organ transplant.

35
Balanced living and gratitude

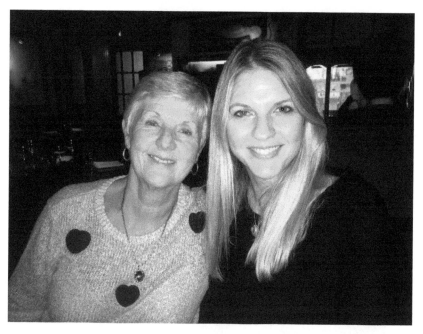

Mum and I celebrating our fifth 'kidney-versary' over some dinner.

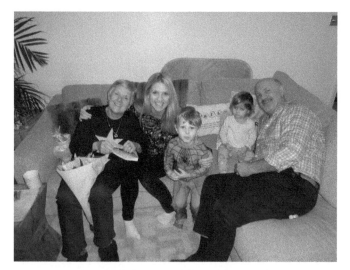

*Mum, Dad, George and Rosealin at our house
celebrating our seven-year 'kidney-versary'.*

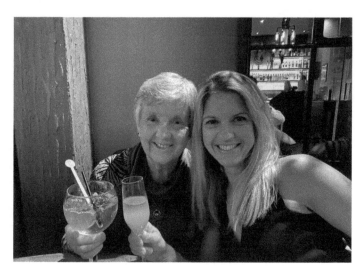

*Mum and I at our nine-year 'kidney-versary',
celebrating with a cocktail over dinner in Beckenham.*

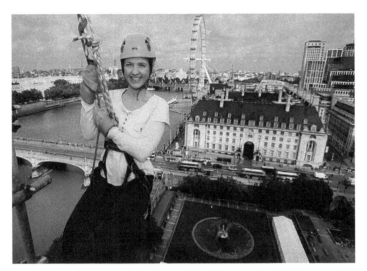

September 2021. Commencing an abseil 160 feet down St Thomas' Hospital while raising money for Guy's and St Thomas' Charity.

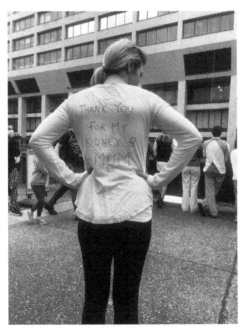

My personalised T-shirt for the Guy's and St Thomas' Charity abseil.

WORK–LIFE BALANCE WITH THE CHILDREN has always been such a priority of mine, and I have been extremely fortunate to have found it. I love being an osteopath and Pilates instructor. More recently I have gone on to do some ad hoc clinical tutoring at one of the osteopathy universities, which has been such fun and a new adventure.

Exercise continues to be an important aspect of my health. I know how important cardiovascular fitness is to manage my blood pressure, which is paramount in managing the health and function of my transplanted kidney. Reformer Pilates classes, yoga, walking and cycling are my go-to forms of exercise as often as possible.

It's amazing how selfless you become once starting a family. The children always take priority. But as they have got a little older (as I write this, Rosa is five and George is seven), I am finding more time to keep my health in check, to exercise and to do things I have an interest in.

For women who have CKD and are thinking about starting a family, it's a decision that takes some thought. Each person's situation is different but having pre-pregnancy counselling with specialists in nephrology as well as in obstetrics can really help you decide what may be the best decision for you.

Fortunately, there is research going on all the time, and a new study is about to begin at King's College Hospital that will examine the issue of fertility in women who have kidney disease.

Our kidney anniversary

Every year since receiving my kidney transplant from Mum, we have an extra celebration. We have dinner with close family, and I thank them for all they did during that time and still do for me, especially Mum. We celebrate the continued success of the transplant, give thanks for the medical team at Guy's Hospital and reflect on the wonderful care Mum and I received while we were hospitalised. We always take a photo of Mum and I to mark this wonderful occasion, the 'gift of another life' celebration.

Guy's and St Thomas' Hospital Charity

My gratitude towards Guy's and St Thomas' Hospital has never wavered, and I have continued to find ways of raising funds to benefit its charity.

Just before each of our children was born, we asked patients to try and guess the weight of the baby, with the winner getting a free treatment at the clinic! Each time, we managed to raise a few hundred pounds.

The most recent challenge I undertook was an abseil off the top of St Thomas' Hospital. That first step off was petrifying, but I felt incredible by the time I reached the bottom. I managed to raise over £500 from generous donations made by family, loved ones, friends and patients.

Thank you again, everyone!

36
CKD support resources

Social media and community groups

Since going through this 'life adventure' I have become interested in reaching out to others who have also experienced organ donation, especially women who have then gone on to have children.

I stumbled across the organisation Transplant Pregnancy Registry International, founded in America. This is an ongoing research study focusing on the effects of pregnancy on transplant recipients and the effects of immunosuppressive medication on fertility and pregnancy outcomes. It has lots of free resources including access to peer-reviewed publications on all different organ transplantations and pregnancy, including kidney and breastfeeding while on immunosuppressant medication. It has a very active page on Facebook. This is a great place to start if you're trying to decide whether to start a family after organ donation.

There is also a Facebook page titled 'Pregnancy and motherhood and organ transplant', which has 3.2 thousand members. This could be a useful resource for those who are pregnant or wanting to conceive with a transplant, or even those considering pregnancy prior to having a transplant. Unfortunately, I did not access this page until after having both my children, but I have contributed by answering questions that have been put to the community of members.

The National Kidney Federation has a fantastic website with real information about kidney conditions. It also enables patients to get in touch with one another. There are three thousand members on its social media page, and the website provides a great opportunity to be part of a community by sharing stories and asking questions. It puts out a seasonal publication called *Kidney Life Magazine*, which features helpful articles on various topics related to kidney disease and real-life stories from kidney patients. There is also a helpful three-part publication written by a renal surgeon, detailing the stages of a transplant. This is a national organisation, founded back in 1979, whereby the forty-nine independent kidney patient associations came together as the controlling council to campaign for improvements to renal provision and treatment along with being a national patient support service. It also offers a free helpline, taking calls from patients, carers and healthcare professionals. I never knew about this until after my transplant! If I had, I believe this resource may have provided me with some much-needed support from others going through the same thing.

Kidney Beam, in partnership with King's College Hospital, is a fantastic resource that was set up during the COVID-19 pandemic for kidney patients. It is an online platform that has live exercise classes and progressive pre-recorded exercise programmes on it, along with specialist wellbeing videos. The site is hosted by kidney professionals including renal physiotherapists, dieticians and counsellors from different NHS trusts. There are also people living with kidney disease performing some of the exercise programmes too. This is a great resource that has been funded by Kidney Research UK, with collaboration from charities such as Kidney

Care UK, National Kidney Federation and UK Kidney Association. Since its launch in 2020, almost two thousand people have signed up. The site is being used to research its effect on health and wellbeing for kidney patients and to hopefully build a case for NHS commissioning. It is free for all kidney patients.

Kidney Care UK is another charity dedicated to helping all those living with kidney disease. It provides kidney patients with emotional, practical and financial help if required. It also has a free seasonal magazine called *Kidney Matters*, which includes articles about latest research, developments in care, patients' stories and charity news.

Kidney Research UK is a British charity that strives to find ways to prevent kidney disease, educate to try to slow progression and help research how to repair kidney damage and find ways of improving treatment. It is working with others to put kidney disease on the UK's health agenda.

The UK Kidney Association is the leading professional body supporting professionals in the delivery of kidney care and research. There are some other smaller UK-based kidney charities: Global Kidney Foundation, Kidneys for Life and The Kidney Fund.

The last, but not least, resource I want to highlight is a fantastic podcast called *Diary of a Kidney Warrior* by Dee Moore. Dee has stage 4 CKD and since August 2020 has interviewed lots of guests exploring all aspects of kidney disease, chronic illness and health. Guests include other kidney patients, renal nurses, psychologists, consultants, dieticians and more. This podcast is for any kidney patient or family member or friend of a kidney patient who may want to learn more about kidney disease. This is well worth a listen.

Professional support

Chapter 6

Kidney Care UK diet information: www.kidneycareuk.org/ about-kidney-health/living-kidney-disease/kidney-kitchen/diet-information-and-advice

Chapter 7

Amanda Reuter: Better Health – Naturally Ltd
Goudhurst Kent
Tel: 01580 212340

Chapter 22

NHS Prescription Prepayment Certificate:
www.services.nhsbsa.nhs.uk/buy-prescription-prepayment-certificate/start

Chapter 30

Janice Champion: www.janice-champion.co.uk

EPI-NO device: www.epi-no.co.uk

Chapter 32

Kate Bramham's paper on breastfeeding and tacrolimus:
www.pubmed.ncbi.nlm.nih.gov/23349333

National Childcare Trust (NCT): www.nct.org.uk

Chapter 36

Transplant Pregnancy Registry International: www.transplantpregnancyregistry.org

National Kidney Federation: www.kidney.org.uk

Kidney Beam : www.beamfeelgood.com/kidney-disease

Kidney Care UK: www.kidneycareuk.org

UK Kidney Association: www.ukkidney.org

Global Kidney Foundation: www.gkf.org.uk

Kidneys for Life: www.kidneysforlife.org

The Kidney Fund: www.kidneyfund.org.uk

Dee Moore's *Diary of a Kidney Warrior*: www.youtube.com/watch?v=VzxAsd4p3GM

Afterword

HEARING STORIES FROM OTHERS with CKD has helped me to feel less isolated and to know that there are always people out there who are less fortunate than I am. This stark realisation really helps me gain perspective when dealing with any situation.

I hope this book about my journey thus far helps give those with CKD the encouragement to go out and fill their life with fun and adventure. The diagnosis may be daunting, but with adequate support, you can still live, not merely survive. I know at some point in my life that things will no doubt change, and my sixty-eight-year-old transplanted kidney may start to fail. I am ever hopeful that with every passing year, more medical interventions and treatment options will be discovered. If and when the time comes, maybe I'll be lucky enough to have another successful transplant!

Waking up being mindfully grateful to be alive every morning is a habit I have gotten into. Filling my life with positive experiences and helping others is what seems to fill my cup. If this book helps just one person on their journey, it has been well worth writing.

Thank you for reading.

Acknowledgements

I HAVE MUCH GRATITUDE TO EXPRESS. Firstly, the incredible NHS staff especially the renal doctors and nurses for diagnosing me, treating me and continuing to care and support me.

I know this book would not have been written and completed if it wasn't for my super encouraging husband, Tim. Thank you so much for your love and support. You are my rock.

Thank you to Guadalupe Molina (Lu), a fellow kidney transplant recipient who helped with the editing stage, highlighting my overzealous use of exclamation marks, one of which I still managed to keep in the title. Thanks also to Michele Moore who copyedited my draft and gave me such encouraging and enthusiastic feedback, helping to build my confidence as a first-time author. Thanks, too, to the team at Jessica Kate Brown Publications for their efforts in formatting and proofreading to get the book ready to publish. Thanks to Neal Manning, a talented graphic designer at Papercuts and Pixels, for the cover design.

I would like to dedicate this book to just a few of the many people in my life including close friends and family whose love and support made this book possible:

My wonderfully supportive family, especially my parents, who are always there for me no matter what.

My one-in-a-million Auntie Lisa, who is my very own personal 'therapist', angel in disguise and very best friend.

My two beautiful, kind and loving children, George and Rosealin, who I love with my whole heart.

And lastly...

My selfless, loving mother. Thanks for my kidney, Mum!

Milton Keynes UK
Ingram Content Group UK Ltd.
UKHW022047250923
429373UK00011B/131